Physical Intelligence

Dr Tom Smith has been writing since 1977, after spending six years in general practice and seven years in medical research. He wrote the 'Doctor, Doctor' column in *The Guardian* on Saturdays, and has written three humorous books, *Doctor, Have You Got a Minute?*, *A Seaside Practice* and *Going Loco*, all published by Short Books. His other books for Sheldon Press include *Heart Attacks: Prevent and Survive*, *Living with Alzheimer's Disease*, *Overcoming Back Pain*, *Coping with Bowel Cancer*, *Coping with Heartburn and Reflux*, *Coping with Age-related Memory Loss*, *101 Questions to Ask Your Doctor*, *How to Get the Best from Your Doctor*, *Coping with Kidney Disease*, *Osteoporosis: Prevent and Treat*, *Coping Successfully with Prostate Cancer* and *Reducing Your Risk of Dementia*.

Overcoming Common Problems Series

Selected titles

A full list of titles is available from Sheldon Press,
36 Causton Street, London SW1P 4ST and on our website at
www.sheldonpress.co.uk

101 Questions to Ask Your Doctor
Dr Tom Smith

Asperger Syndrome in Adults
Dr Ruth Searle

The Assertiveness Handbook
Mary Hartley

Assertiveness: Step by Step
Dr Windy Dryden and Daniel Constantinou

Backache: What you need to know
Dr David Delvin

Birth Over 35
Sheila Kitzinger

Body Language: What you need to know
David Cohen

Breast Cancer: Your treatment choices
Dr Terry Priestman

Bulimia, Binge-eating and their Treatment
Professor J. Hubert Lacey, Dr Bryony Bamford
and Amy Brown

The Cancer Survivor's Handbook
Dr Terry Priestman

The Chronic Pain Diet Book
Neville Shone

Cider Vinegar
Margaret Hills

Coeliac Disease: What you need to know
Alex Gazzola

**Coping Successfully with Chronic Illness:
Your healing plan**
Neville Shone

Coping Successfully with Pain
Neville Shone

Coping Successfully with Prostate Cancer
Dr Tom Smith

Coping Successfully with Shyness
Margaret Oakes, Professor Robert Bor and
Dr Carina Eriksen

Coping Successfully with Ulcerative Colitis
Peter Cartwright

Coping Successfully with Varicose Veins
Christine Craggs-Hinton

Coping Successfully with Your Hiatus Hernia
Dr Tom Smith

Coping When Your Child Has Cerebral Palsy
Jill Eckersley

Coping with Anaemia
Dr Tom Smith

Coping with Asthma in Adults
Mark Greener

**Coping with Birth Trauma and Postnatal
Depression**
Lucy Jolin

Coping with Bronchitis and Emphysema
Dr Tom Smith

Coping with Candida
Shirley Trickett

Coping with Chemotherapy
Dr Terry Priestman

Coping with Chronic Fatigue
Trudie Chalder

Coping with Coeliac Disease
Karen Brody

Coping with Diverticulitis
Peter Cartwright

Coping with Drug Problems in the Family
Lucy Jolin

Coping with Dyspraxia
Jill Eckersley

Coping with Early-onset Dementia
Jill Eckersley

Coping with Eating Disorders and Body Image
Christine Craggs-Hinton

Coping with Epilepsy
Dr Pamela Crawford and Fiona Marshall

Coping with Gout
Christine Craggs-Hinton

Coping with Guilt
Dr Windy Dryden

Coping with Headaches and Migraine
Alison Frith

Coping with Heartburn and Reflux
Dr Tom Smith

Coping with Life after Stroke
Dr Mareeni Raymond

**Coping with Life's Challenges: Moving on
from adversity**
Dr Windy Dryden

Overcoming Common Problems Series

Coping with Liver Disease
Mark Greener

Coping with Manipulation: When others
blame you for their feelings
Dr Windy Dryden

Coping with Obsessive Compulsive Disorder
Professor Kevin Gournay, Rachel Piper
and Professor Paul Rogers

Coping with Phobias and Panic
Professor Kevin Gournay

Coping with PMS
Dr Farah Ahmed and Dr Emma Cordle

Coping with Polycystic Ovary Syndrome
Christine Craggs-Hinton

Coping with the Psychological Effects
of Cancer
Professor Robert Bor, Dr Carina Eriksen
and Ceilidh Stapelkamp

Coping with Radiotherapy
Dr Terry Priestman

Coping with Snoring and Sleep Apnoea
Jill Eckersley

Coping with Stomach Ulcers
Dr Tom Smith

Coping with Suicide
Maggie Helen

Coping with Type 2 Diabetes
Susan Elliot-Wright

Depressive Illness: The curse of the strong
Dr Tim Cantopher

The Diabetes Healing Diet
Mark Greener and Christine Craggs-Hinton

Dying for a Drink
Dr Tim Cantopher

Dynamic Breathing: How to manage
your asthma
Dinah Bradley and Tania Clifton-Smith

The Empathy Trap: Understanding
Antisocial Personalities
Dr Jane McGregor and Tim McGregor

Epilepsy: Complementary and alternative
treatments
Dr Sallie Baxendale

The Fibromyalgia Healing Diet
Christine Craggs-Hinton

Fibromyalgia: Your Treatment Guide
Christine Craggs-Hinton

Free Yourself from Depression
Colin and Margaret Sutherland

A Guide to Anger Management
Mary Hartley

Hay Fever: How to beat it
Dr Paul Carson

The Heart Attack Survival Guide
Mark Greener

Helping Children Cope with Grief
Rosemary Wells

How to Beat Worry and Stress
Dr David Delvin

How to Come Out of Your Comfort Zone
Dr Windy Dryden

How to Develop Inner Strength
Dr Windy Dryden

How to Eat Well When You Have Cancer
Jane Freeman

How to Live with a Control Freak
Barbara Baker

How to Lower Your Blood Pressure:
And keep it down
Christine Craggs-Hinton

How to Manage Chronic Fatigue
Christine Craggs-Hinton

The IBS Healing Plan
Theresa Cheung

Let's Stay Together: A guide to lasting
relationships
Jane Butterworth

Living with Angina
Dr Tom Smith

Living with Asperger Syndrome
Dr Joan Gomez

Living with Autism
Fiona Marshall

Living with Bipolar Disorder
Dr Neel Burton

Living with Complicated Grief
Professor Craig A. White

Living with Crohn's Disease
Dr Joan Gomez

Living with Eczema
Jill Eckersley

Living with Fibromyalgia
Christine Craggs-Hinton

Living with Gluten Intolerance
Jane Feinmann

Living with IBS
Nuno Ferreira and David T. Gillanders

Living with Loss and Grief
Julia Tugendhat

Living with Osteoarthritis
Dr Patricia Gilbert

Living with Physical Disability
and Amputation
Dr Keren Fisher

Living with Rheumatoid Arthritis
Philippa Pigache

Overcoming Common Problems Series

Overcoming Common Problems

Physical Intelligence
How to take charge of your weight

DR TOM SMITH

sheldon PRESS

First published in Great Britain in 2013

Sheldon Press
36 Causton Street
London SW1P 4ST
www.sheldonpress.co.uk

British Library Cataloguing-in-Publication Data
A catalogue record for this book is available from the British Library

ISBN 978–1–84709–281–6
eBook ISBN 978–1–84709–282–3

Typeset by Caroline Waldron, Wirral, Cheshire
First printed in Great Britain by Ashford Colour Press
Subsequently digitally printed in Great Britain

Produced on paper from sustainable forests

To the members of the Medical Journalists' Association, who have provided immense help and friendship over many years, especially those who have worked on The Lancet, British Medical Journal *and* New Scientist, *the unbiased reporting and analysis of which have provided me with so much information that I could trust. This book's foundation lies in the professionalism of this elite group of dedicated followers of science and medicine.*

Contents

Preface

The following few quotes illustrate themes relevant to the content of this book. They will make sense as you read on!

Thou seest I have more flesh than another man, therefore more frailty.

> Falstaff to Prince Hal, Act 3, Scene 3,
> *Henry V, Part I*, William Shakespeare, 1604

Although obesity can cause health problems, it does not necessarily make people feel worse in the absence of such problems.

Educational interventions are unlikely to work because obese people aren't unhappy enough to lose weight.

> Paul Dolan and Georgios Kavetsos,
> *British Medical Journal*, 2012

What have we been doing in the last 400 years? Have we forgotten Falstaff?

Obesity is not only caused by how much we eat or drink. Our chances of being obese are also affected by factors like whether we have easy access to affordable fruit, vegetables, and other healthy foods and if it is safe to let our kids play outside. That's why a government focus on personal choice alone is at best a red herring and at worst a dereliction of duty for everyone's health.

> Zosia Kmietowicz, *British Medical Journal*, 2013

I'm on your side, Zosia.

In 2012, 1632 British doctors responded to the question, 'What is more important to you – the taste of food or how healthy it is?'

Some 58.5 per cent voted for taste. I'm on your side, too, doctors. I would have done the same.

Introduction

Connections. Our family used to play this game when I was a child. We were given a list of seemingly unconnected subjects and drove ourselves mad trying to link them. My father was a school-teacher, which probably explains our odd family source of amusement, and it was he who devised the lists. It also explains why I didn't follow in his footsteps. In this book, however, I'm reverting to family type. I'm imposing a game on you. Here is a list of things that I want you to connect.

- prehistoric man
- 17,000 Whitehall civil servants
- 48,000 Swedish women
- Pima Indians of Arizona
- South Pacific islanders
- Messrs Atkins, Hay and Dukan
- the Cambridge diet
- the Hairy Bikers
- those old school photographs, in which the pupils sat around in a huge semi-circle several rows deep
- today's schoolchildren
- two Wembley international football matches – one between England and Scotland in 1967 and one between England and Sweden in 2005
- two substances called ghrelin and leptin
- Charlie Walduck of Barrow-in-Furness.

Maybe you are halfway there, but, please, if you are curious, read on.

This is a book on understanding our physiology – the ways in which our bodies work – and how modern life almost necessarily alters it in subtle ways that can lead to our becoming overweight and unhealthy. At this point, you may be starting to yawn, wondering 'Do I really want to read yet another book on weight gain and loss?'

I'd like to think that this one is different from the others. It is based on the premise that when we truly understand how our bodies work, we can form an intelligent approach to keeping normally fit and healthy. All the above connections have something to tell us about that and they are peculiarly relevant to our lives today.

There are so many books on diets and exercise advice for people who are anything from a little overweight to frankly obese that, at first sight, yet another one is superfluous. You are entitled to ask for it to have a different, perhaps unique, viewpoint, a theme that would mark it out from its competitors – and make obvious sense. So, how about one that is based entirely on logic and reason, with advice that stems from evidence-based research and peer-reviewed publications in high-quality medical and scientific journals?

Add to that a little history (and prehistory) and a few case histories from the books of many family doctors, plus even a touch of humour. Let me give you just a few examples. One of my own stories relating to patient–doctor cooperation and confrontation is that of a woman who got so angry with me for suggesting that her daughter needed to lose weight (she was a 14-year-old weighing 15 stone, which is 95 kg or 210 lbs), she threw a bucket of window-cleaning water over me! There was also the sad 42-year-old man weighing 37 stone (235 kg or 518 lbs) who needed a forklift truck to get him out of the house to the ambulance and the jolly, happily healthy and physically fit 18-year-old girl (she rode a Clydesdale horse to work every day) who was so overweight that she didn't know she was pregnant until she went into labour.

These are all extreme examples, but they illustrate points that need to be explained, such as the defensive anger people feel when confronted with the need to do something about their, or their child's, health. There is the sense of hopelessness that they feel, so they just continue on an always worsening upward weight spiral. There are the complications that being overweight can bring, even when they are young.

How have these people reached these crises in their lives? In the past, they would have been looked on as extreme. I am occasionally asked to talk to primary school children about healthy living. During these talks I show them my old school photograph. In it there are more than 400 boys, aged from 11 to 18 and around 30 teachers. I ask today's kids what they find odd about the photo-graph. They talk about the school uniform, the short trousers the younger boys have on, the fact that there are no girls . . . but they don't see the real difference from today. When I point out that there is not a single overweight person, boy or adult, in the whole picture, they are astonished.

When I started these talks, in the late noughties, showing the photograph raised difficult issues that I hadn't expected, but should have foreseen. At that time, among every class of children in my audiences of 8 to 11-year-olds, there were two or three who were already considerably overweight or even classifiable as obese. Even worse, perhaps, around a third of their teachers were notice-ably overweight, too.

It was difficult, of course, because, by highlighting the difference between my generation and theirs, I was inadvertently adding to the possible abuse – verbal and even physical – that 'fat' (I use the word here because that's what their peers used) children experi-enced daily from their classmates. The odd fat teacher might not have felt comfortable about it either. So, I had to go on to try and explain what had happened in the intervening years to our popu-lation without making the 'outliers' feel even more antagonized than they already were.

I find my talks to schoolchildren are much easier now. I don't know if my more recent experience would be reflected throughout the UK, but in our area of rural South West Scotland, the children, their families and their teachers appear to have 'got the message'. I have been to primary schools where there is no bullying of fatter children – because there are none. The children, boys and girls, are the same shape as their grandparents were at the same age.

The difference from five years ago? The schools have put in place a sensible, well-thought-out physical exercise programme that the children all enjoy – and not just a PE lesson twice a week. They enjoy being active, even sporty, and the difference this makes shows. The teachers take part, too. They are just as enthusiastic as their little charges and it shows in their waistlines, too. One teacher in her thirties has shed 4 stone in three years (over 25 kilograms) and puts the loss down entirely to her new schooltime activities – she hasn't changed her lifestyle in any other way.

Initially, when the schools began to take the health message seriously, there were teething problems. The idea, of course, was not simply to help the children generally to become physically fitter, but to try and target those who were overweight and help them adopt lifestyle changes that would help them become slimmer naturally. We came up against unforeseen challenges. Parents would send their children to school with a note asking that they be excused from the exercise classes because they made them breathless or they didn't want to undress down to their gym kit in front of the others or it made them unhappy and ashamed because they couldn't keep up with the others. There were even notes claiming (falsely of course) that their doctors had advised them their children were not fit enough to attend the exercise periods – one was purportedly from me!

Parents (usually overweight themselves) would become aggressive towards the teachers when a note was sent back refusing to accede to these requests. It wasn't an easy start to the new regime, but the exercise programme eventually won through. It succeeded not because of a change in the parents' attitudes, but because the overweight children found, to their own astonishment, that they began to enjoy the games and sports. The boys started to enjoy the dancing and the girls the football. Stereotypes fell away into the past and excess weight was lost happily and faster than anyone had hoped.

The parents of the heavier children were slower to come round to the new lifestyle than their children. We (that is, the teachers and I) presumed that most of them were probably desperate to come off what they saw as an inevitable path towards an even heavier future but didn't know how. They would have tried all the diets and the exercises (though most would not have persisted with the exercises for long enough), reading about them in magazines and so on, yet always failed to maintain what weight loss they had achieved on them. They also saw – unhappily, guiltily and with a considerable sense of shame – their children turning out the same way and, if they failed, how could their children succeed?

So, my first message to them as well as you is that nothing is simple about being overweight or obese. If you are, you must first jettison any shame or blame you feel for your condition – neither response is helpful and will only make it more difficult to reverse the situation. You need to know why some people become overweight and others don't.

You will have noticed that, so far, I haven't mentioned changing eating habits to lose weight: I have only mentioned exercise. That's because the amount we eat plays only a secondary part in the process of the trail from being a normal weight to being overweight to being obese. Of course, gluttony leads to obesity, but where does the drive to eat more and more, and exercise less and less, come from? Understanding that first process is key to how we approach the solution to the problem of becoming at first overweight, then, frankly, obese, then morbidly so. Why it happens to some people and not to others is nothing to do with laziness or gluttony, but, rather, with our particular body chemistry and I will spell out these inherited differences plainly, in lay language, in the first two chapters.

Crucial to this understanding is how we explain hunger. Hours after a meal, cells in the lining of the upper part of our stomachs and in our pancreas start to secrete a hormone called ghrelin into our bloodstream. This reaches the brain, which reacts by making us feel hungry. As we eat in response to this feeling, we set off a 'feedback' mechanism to reduce our appetite. Ghrelin levels fall and our fat cells in our tissues begin to secrete an opposing hormone, leptin, which curbs hunger. In normal circumstances, almost precisely 20 minutes after we start to eat, we have lost our feeling of hunger completely – regardless of how much we have eaten in that time! So, if we eat slowly and moderate our mouthfuls in those 20 minutes, we will take in far less food than if we gobble up our food and take in more of it as a result.

If this message is new to you, it certainly isn't new to the electronics industry. The Consumer Electronics Show, held in Las Vegas annually, is where the giants of electronic wizardry show off their new products. The agreed highlight of the 2013 exhibition – it featured in several UK television shows, including primetime news – was the HAPIfork™. This surprising piece of cutlery has a handle that vibrates and flashes a light when you are using it too often – in other words, eating too fast. You can even download an analysis of your chewing data and share it with your Facebook or

YouTube friends. It is at least a step in the right direction in that it highlights fast eating as being one of factors leading to obesity.

So, eating slowly is one key to eating less. There do seem to be people, however, who don't have an effective leptin response, so they still feel hungry after 20 minutes (we will look at this in a little more detail in Chapter 5). Much research has been devoted to ghrelin, leptin and similar chemicals and in Chapter 5 I will explain how they can influence obesity in enough detail to inform, but not confuse, you. As you can imagine, one avenue of research into obesity has concentrated on drugs that might suppress appetite using leptin or anti-ghrelin-like chemicals.

How much you eat is probably more important than what you eat, despite all the magazine articles about diets specifically designed to help men and women lose weight. Low-carb diets, low-fat diets, high-protein diets, high-fibre diets, very low-calorie diets – they are all advocated with little evidence that any of them are effective (except during the very short times people can tolerate them for) – and all of them have their dangers. One crucial example is the Atkins diet, which advocates that we should eat very little carbohydrate and loads of protein. It has plenty of devotees. They possibly haven't read the *British Medical Journal*'s editorial and a report on a study that monitored 43,396 Swedish women for an average of 15.7 years (Floegel and Pischon, 2012, and Lagiou et al., 2012, respectively). The study showed conclusively that an Atkins-like diet increased their chances of developing serious heart disease, and dying from it, by 62 per cent over women who just ate a normal diet. Those on the Atkins-like diet became thinner, but put themselves at this much higher risk of heart attack and stroke. For 'Atkins' also read Hay, Dukan and Cambridge, in that they restrict the variety of foods you eat, so face the same problems and probable outcomes.

Everyone surely knows that there are three basic forms of material that make up our food – fats, carbohydrates and proteins. Fewer people know that fats and sugars are virtually interchangeable. Fats convert into carbohydrates (mainly glucose), while carbohydrates (starches and sugars) convert freely into fats. So a low-fat, high-starch food can produce as much body fat as a high-fat, low-sugar food.

Proteins are different in that, after digestion, they are split into amino acids – the building blocks of our tissues and organs. This fact formed the basis of the Atkins diet – it being proposed that eating a lot of protein-rich food would not lead to excess fat deposits. If we eat more protein than we need, though, it, too, can be turned into potentially lethal fatty deposits in the blood vessel walls in the heart and brain. So, a lot has to be explained about foods and how we change them into the substances we need to keep healthy, which I will do in Chapter 1.

1

We hunter-gatherers

How has this system of processing foods in our bodies evolved? We can't escape the fact that we are all still, physically, hunter-gatherers, even though most of our ancestors swapped this behaviour for agriculture around 10,000–20,000 years ago.

As hunter-gatherers, both men and women would roam around 20 or more miles a day until they had found enough food to return to their primitive shelters or caves and eat it all. They ate until they were satiated, then slept. They might have rested for a day or two before they were so hungry again that they went on another hunting or foraging trip. The problem was that there were times when they could hardly find enough food and other times when there was a glut. The evidence suggests that modern humans have been around for at least 80,000 years and maybe for as long as 2 million years and for most of this time we were beset by such feast or famine situations. We starved until we could find enough food · for ourselves and our kin, then we ate our full and slept it off until we were hungry again.

Doing this for so long, our body chemistry and physiology (our dynamic bodily systems) had to adapt to the seesawing in the supply of food to be digested. During the glut periods, our ancestors stored any excess of digested foods as fat, to be called on when they were starving. Evolution has ensured that this has become an extremely efficient system, converting any extra food into fat to be used for energy when there is no food to be found. The 10,000 or so years since most of us gave up hunter-gathering for primitive, then more sophisticated, farming, has not been enough time for our bodies to have changed to another system of energy storage. Alas, we are still exceptionally well programmed to accumulate fat in the tissues under our skin and around our gut and, sadly, for many of us, in the lining of our blood vessels and heart.

Today, of course, no one in the developed world (provided we are not fighting wars) starves because food is freely available to us every day, all year round. Nor do we have to travel marathon distances on foot to collect it. On the hunter-gatherer scale, we don't need to exert ourselves to find and eat our food and we have plenty of it around us to assuage any fleeting instances of hunger. So, we keep converting the food that we eat but don't need for energy purposes into fat storage. Over days, weeks and years these deposits accumulate into excess weight that is very difficult to burn off without starving ourselves or becoming the equivalent of a hunter-gatherer. Remember, hunter gathering involves spending at least five hours every day on the hoof, often breaking into a run to catch a small mammal or avoid a much bigger one with long and sharp teeth that is also practising, very efficiently, the art of hunter-gathering.

If you have any doubts about this, spend a little time with the Pima Indians. You don't have to go back thousands of years for the proof of what I've been describing: we have examples of people this happened to in the twentieth century.

The Pima live in the Gila River area of Arizona, in the USA. They happily combined basic farming and hunting, as their ancestors had done since they settled in the area more than 2000 years ago. Over many years, they engineered irrigation systems to allow them to grow fruit, vegetables and cotton. The women were famous for their baskets, so closely woven that they were watertight. The work for both men and women was physically hard, but worthwhile and productive and they were known for their generous hospitality and kindness to anyone passing through their lands.

The happiness ended when American farmers of European origin living further up the river took the Pima's water supply to use on their own fields. Without water, the Pima starved and became poverty-stricken. They needed help from the US government, which gave them what was seen then as nourishing food – largely sugar, processed flour and lard. No longer able to farm or hunt – the lack of water destroyed more than the Pima: it destroyed the wildlife, too – they now were fed without having to exert themselves, with what turned out to be exactly the wrong types of foodstuffs, with the potential to provide them with much more energy than they could ever expend, even if they had remained hunter-gatherers and farmers. As agriculture was no longer an option (there were no more animals to be hunted, not enough wild plants to gather in a land that had reverted to desert and, with the source of their irrigation system stopped, no fields to manage), they sat around, ate much more than they needed and grew fat.

Before this disaster struck, around the end of the nineteenth century, only 15 per cent of the Pima's food was fat – the rest was mainly starch and fibre, with a small amount of animal-based protein. By the middle of the twentieth century, they were getting 40 per cent of their energy from fatty foods.

The Second World War made things much worse for them. The young men joined up and became the first generation of Pima to be immersed in the great American society. Many young men and women moved to cities and their incomes multiplied as they found productive jobs in factories. Most of them returned to their traditional lands after the war, but they brought with them their new lifestyle. No longer did they tolerate the hardships involved in working the land or the government handouts – they wanted more. The change towards a more sedentary and relatively affluent life accelerated and they became even fatter and, to their doctors' surprise at the time (there would have been no surprise today), they developed diabetes.

During this 100 years or so of change for the Arizonan Pima, there was a 'control group' living quietly in the Mexican Sierra Madre mountains. Dr Eric Ravussin and colleagues, who began their study of the Pima in Arizona in 1978, visited them in the early years of this century. The Sierra Madre are hundreds of miles from the Gila River, but they are home to another community of Pima who were found to be genetically the same as their Arizonan cousins. Dr Ravussin and his colleagues examined 35 Sierra Madre Pimas and found them to be slim and healthy. Only three of them had diabetes, which is not very different from what would be expected in any healthy community. The crucial difference between the two 'families' was that the Mexican Pima had never adopted the American lifestyle taken up by their Gila River cousins, but were still small farmers and hunters.

Control groups are crucial to any scientific endeavour – they help to put the conclusions in perspective and this one emphasized that the change in health of the Arizonan Pima was indeed due to the change in lifestyle. The proof that is really needed is to reverse the change in lifestyle, to see if it reverses the ill health. That is where the Pima have triumphed – magnificently.

Ravussin and his colleague's (1994) conclusions were clear. I quote from his study:

> We've learned from this study of the Mexican Pimas that if the Pima Indians of Arizona could return to some of their traditions, including a high degree of physical activity and a diet with less fat and more starch, we might be able to reduce the rate, and surely the severity, of unhealthy weight in most of the population.

Of course, there were difficulties in achieving this as, among the post-war Pima generation, one half had diabetes and 95 per cent of them were seriously overweight. Over the first 30 years of the Pima study, the proof emerged that obesity was for them – and, just as important, for the rest of us – the primary cause of their diabetes. The Pima embraced the studies enthusiastically, as they knew that they were far sicker and dying younger than their forebears. They applied themselves to reversing the change.

One of the first new findings to emerge from the study was that the people, men and women, who were going to put on the most weight as adults started with a distinct disadvantage. Their metabolism – the rate at which they turned over foodstuffs into energy – was slower than in the (relatively small) number of Pima who didn't put on extra weight. The scientists concluded that this slower metabolic rate, when combined with a high-fat diet and an inherited tendency to store more fat more easily, was the cause of what was described as an 'epidemic' of being overweight among the Pima.

In 1962, geneticist James Neel coined the phrase the 'thrifty gene' to explain the Pima's problem. He proposed that, for thousands of years, all populations, not just the Pima, who relied on farming, hunting and fishing for food – in fact, the ancestors of almost all of us (extremely few communities of ancient humans had plentiful food all the time) – had to live with alternating periods of feast and famine. To cope with these wide variations in food supply, most of our ancestors had to develop a thrifty gene that helped them to store fat during the bountiful times so they could use it when the food sources dried up. Those who didn't possess the thrifty gene either died during famines or somehow just managed to get along.

This gene was helpful as long as there were periods of famine, but, once these populations adopted the typical Western lifestyle, with less physical activity, a high-fat diet and access to a constant supply of calories, this gene began to work against them, continuing to store calories in preparation for famine despite there never being one. Thus, scientists think the thrifty gene that once protected people from starvation might also contribute to their retaining unhealthy amounts of fat and developing diabetes.

The young adult Pima of today know all about the thrifty gene, as the case histories on the US's National Institute of Diabetes and Digestive and Kidney Diseases' (NIDDK) website describe in detail (at: <http://diabetes.niddk.nih.gov/dm/pubs/pima/obesity/obesity.htm>). For example, Donna, a 25-year-old, described on the website as a picture of glowing health, was overweight until she was 24. She knew that many members of her immediate family had diabetes, including her grandparents on both sides, but she hadn't really considered that she might have the illness, too. Then she had a blood glucose test and the result shocked her. She joined a friend in walking two miles every day, exercised more and ate less than before. She lost weight and slimmed down where she wanted to and her blood glucose level, initially in the diabetes 'at risk' range, became normal. She now also has plenty of energy to look after her three children.

In 2013, today's Gila River Pima are back to being an industrious agricultural community, looking after orchards of orange trees, pistachios and olives. The 11,000 members of the Gila River Indian Reservation have happily taken part in more than three decades of research that has enormously helped our understanding of how obesity happens, how it often leads to diabetes and how it can be reversed by the whole community cooperating in making lifestyle changes. By striking a balance between what they eat and how much physical work they do, the Pima have not only avoided becoming diabetic, but also have healthier eyes, hearts and kidneys again. They are living longer and are happier than their parents.

The story doesn't end there. Scientists at the NIDDK are still studying the Pima, and their willing subjects have agreed to their work continuing for generations. The Pima have lived around the Gila River for hundreds of years and the present generation of youngsters still marry largely within their community. Dr William Knowler of the NIDDK writes that this has given us a deeper and better understanding of the links between obesity and diabetes. The first 30 years of the study have shown how difficult it is to pinpoint the relative contributions of inheritance and lifestyle to becoming overweight and/or diabetic or not. The researchers have established, however, that avoiding obesity by enjoying physical activity and eating wisely (foods rich in fibre in the proper amounts are the salient points for the Pima) will at least delay diabetes and may prevent it altogether. This is true even for people whose genetic make-up renders them particularly susceptible to developing the disease. The study has also showed that some 80 per cent of people with Type 2 diabetes are overweight and that finding applies to all of us, not just the Pima.

The Pima aren't the only group to have been so affected. The South Pacific islanders have been faced with similar problems – switching from being fishing communities to modern consumers in the space of a few decades. Like the Pima, they, too, have paid the price in obesity, high blood pressure, diabetes and early death from heart attack and stroke. Sadly, they haven't yet followed the example of the Pima and turned things around.

The Finns faced a different problem. In North Karelia, the northernmost province of Finland, the people were highly dependent on dairy products for their main source of food. North Karelians were generally not obviously obese, but most were overweight. In the 1960s, the district was flagged up as, by far, the least healthy in Finland, with the highest rates of stroke and heart attacks in the world.

The Finnish Health Service started a countrywide policy of health education, informing people as to how to eat better and reduce their dependency on animal fats and proteins, and the results have been astonishing. Like the Pima, the North Karelians made the sensible choice and their illness and death rates fell steeply. Now they are among the healthiest people in Europe.

Easy, isn't it? All we have to do to keep healthy is eat wisely and not overindulge and exercise. If the Pima and the Karelians can do it, why not us? That appears to be the message. If that was all we needed to know and put into practice, however, I could finish this book here and everyone would be happy, slim and fit. We all know that life isn't like that. It is not so easy to control our eating and drinking and it is even harder to follow a programme of exercise that will make, then keep, you fit and well. (The two aren't actually the same.)

So, the main aim of the next two chapters is to persuade you to change your life for the better, based on knowledge rather than guesswork and tradition. Another aim is to show you all the advantages for your future health that exercise and healthy eating bring. You may be surprised – exercise isn't just about getting yourself a six-pack and wise eating isn't all about reducing the size of your waist.

We will start with exercise, but first I want to return you to the first few paragraphs of the Introduction. Remember, I asked what linked a series of apparently unconnected subjects, such as Swedish women and old school photographs? I've mentioned most of the others, too, in the last few pages. The British civil servants appear later, but I've left my two favourites for the end of this chapter – the Hairy Bikers and Charlie Walduck. They are excellent examples for anyone with a severe weight problem.

I hugely enjoy the Hairy Bikers' programmes on British television. They are two happy and very funny lads from the north-east of England who travel around showing off their culinary skills, and challenging local chefs to match them in creating wonderful meals, celebrating recipes passed down the generations and so on. They are bearded, hence the 'Hairy', and they get around on motorcycles, hence the 'Bikers'. They were also very heavy. They won't mind me describing them as being, at the start of 2012, around 30 per cent overweight. They needed to lose 4 or 5 stone (25 to 32 kg or 56 to 70 lbs) to bring themselves into a normal weight range.

Throughout 2012, they abandoned their motorcycles and took to bicycles, becoming the Hairy Dieters. They still conjured up appetising and generous meals for their audiences and, apparently, continued to wolf them down themselves, but they lost weight – spectacularly so. With each programme they were visibly lighter and the weight loss was almost entirely to do with their conversion to pedal power. In effect, they became 'hunters' again and their physiques responded. In the meantime, their show changed, too. From being a standard cookery programme that delighted in the wide variety of regional foods throughout Britain, the Bikers turned it into one that also pushed, ever so gently, the health message, showing how anyone who is overweight or frankly obese can lose their excess weight without missing out on enjoying the good things in life.

What about Charlie Walduck? Charlie featured in the British national press in 2012. At 44 years old he weighed 51 stone (324 kg or 714 lbs). It finally got through to him, with the help of Dr Chris Steele, the expert medical journalist who appears regularly on the British television show *This Morning*, that he would die soon if he did not change his life. Chris didn't think Charlie would manage the change without the help of stomach (bariatric) surgery (about which more later).

I must say, looking at photographs of the 51-stone Charlie, I would have agreed with Chris at the time, but Charlie made it without having an operation. Amazingly, he managed to lose almost four-fifths of his bodyweight by beginning to exercise and eating less. It wasn't easy to start exercising again for someone so heavy, but he did so. Nor did he find it easy to limit himself to one pie instead of his former six at a time, but, when he reached 16 stone (102 kg, 224 lbs), he was able to run marathons – yes, marathons, not just half marathons.

Presumably Charlie has had to have some of the excess skin removed, but, apart from that, he hasn't needed medical intervention and he looks great. Not surprisingly, he spends his time helping others who have been crippled by their obesity. If anyone is an archetypal and successful hunter-gatherer, it is Charlie Walduck.

By now you must be getting the strong message that keeping active, rather than going on a weird diet, is the key to achieving a normal shape, but exercise is much more than simply a way to lose weight. It offers you many more advantages in terms of better health, some of which may surprise you. The next chapter describes what these are.

2

Exercise intelligence

Many doctor friends of mine drop their titles when they are on holiday. They travel incognito, preferring not to get involved in conversations about personal health (or, more usually, ill health) that become inevitable when the secret of their professional life is discovered. I understand and respect their feelings, as they need a complete break from the hard work and commitment of being a doctor.

I have taken a different approach. I have not been in full-time practice for more than 30 years. More than half my time has been taken up with writing – books and for journals and newspapers– so I have had the massive privilege of practising medicine part-time. I therefore don't feel the need to escape from what can seem an all-consuming experience if you are a doctor all day, every day. So, when I travel, I don't hide my profession. It means that sometimes I have had to step up to the plate when needed, but I can still enjoy talking about health and medicine with my fellow travellers rather than see it as a chore. This readiness to talk about health has created for me a ripe source of material for my books, including this one.

From time to time my wife and I have enjoyed going on cruises – an experience that I suspect more than any other pastime helps you to understand the difference between those who embrace exercise and those who do not. On one cruise – to and from Los Angeles, taking in the Hawaiian islands on the way – we were amazed by the number of grossly obese fellow passengers. Around half of them needed wheelchairs or Zimmer frames – the users of the former had become too heavy to walk and the latter were well on their way to the same state. In the dining room in the evenings, the Zimmer frames were lined up like shopping trolleys in a supermarket, rolling backwards and forwards gently with the ocean swell.

It occurred to me that this was like a mass suicide pact, especially as there was no sign that the users of the Zimmer frames and wheelchairs had made any attempt to curb their overeating habits or join the small minority of passengers who, like us, used the gym. When they were not eating in the official dining areas, they were lying motionless in deckchairs, the jacuzzi or inappropriately named 'health spa', blissfully happy, being attended to by the ever-helpful deck staff.

At the opposite end of the scale of this pattern of behaviour was the tragic case of a young woman on the cruise with her devoted parents. Cadaverously thin, she spent her days relentlessly swimming strongly up and down the pool. She was there at 7 a.m. when I was up for a walk round the deck and she was still there at dusk, her mother sitting by the pool's edge, waiting, mostly haplessly, to try and tempt her to eat something at the times when she took a breather. Her obvious anorexia was killing her and her obsession with exercise would only accelerate the process.

The ship's doctor told me that this cruise in particular was burdened more than most by the grossly obese because the American passengers did not need to take a plane to reach the port. Sitting in an aeroplane seat was an impossibility for them, so they chose the one cruise that they could reach by car or train. For the medical and nursing staff, the 15-day journey was hard work. Heart attacks, heart failure, stroke, digestive disorders, diabetic comas, gallbladder spasms and injuries due to falls on deck, out of bed and in the relatively cramped toilets were daily occurrences. Sad to say, the numbers of deaths on each cruise were high.

I liked the ship's doctor. Because I had been listed on the passenger information as a medic, he had sought me out at the welcome party. Having graduated in South Africa and being keen to come to Britain, he was curious to know how our National Health Service worked. We met several times afterwards over coffees and the conversation naturally turned at times to how we might approach the very real problems of obesity – and its opposite.

We eventually agreed that the first step in helping our patients was to get them to understand the role of exercise in their lives, then put it into practice. We agreed the eating problems were probably secondary to that. His role as a ship's doctor, whose patients were fleetingly under his care – they were only there for two weeks – left him feeling hopeless, but he still tried his best.

His attempts at guiding obese 'customers' towards adopting better lifestyles on board had failed miserably: none of them listened. They saw the cruise as the best opportunity in their lives to eat as much as they could for free and be pampered without the need to lift a finger. In particular, he knew of not a single obese customer who had joined the exercise classes in the gym or on deck, despite his best efforts. They might have tried to walk around the track on the top deck, but none of them lasted even a couple of laps (there were 13 laps to a mile) before giving up. They hadn't done so because they were breathless, tired or with pains in their chest; they simply didn't like doing it. Equally, guidance given to the anorexic girl to do less exercise (he, like me, was very worried that she was exercising herself to death) had also fallen on deaf ears.

We pondered together as to why so many people have such distorted attitudes to normal, healthy, physical activity. When and why had they lost that childhood delight in running and jumping, swimming and cycling, playing team games and generally feeling how good it is to be fit and active? What makes them prefer to sit and eat and sleep instead? On the other side of the coin, what makes some exercisers go to the extreme and damage themselves by doing so?

We didn't find answers to these questions, but we did mull over the advantages (and sometimes the disadvantages) of exercise. We resolved to keep in touch and share what we might find in the literature about it. My South African colleague has now left the high seas and is a hardworking general practitioner in the UK. This book is partly the result of those conversations on the Pacific Ocean and I hope he appreciates his hand in it.

Let's start with why he and I agreed that lack of exercise is more important than what we eat in making us fat. When I was a medical student, our lecturer in nutrition told us of an experiment in a 'calorie-controlled' room. I wish I could find the reference to it, but it was many years ago and references weren't my main concern then. Still, I have the gist of it ingrained in my memory.

In the study, in turn, volunteers were kept in a room for a week.

All the subjects were given exactly the same food throughout the week and asked to eat as much as they wished. What was left was measured for energy content so that the researchers could accurately gauge how much they had eaten. The room was maintained at the same comfortable temperature for the week and the energy used to keep it at that temperature was calculated. It is a simple idea – the lower the cost of the energy, the more heat the subject has emitted into the environment and the more physical activity he or she has indulged in. The subjects were weighed at the beginning and the end of their weeks.

The subjects fell into one of two groups – the researchers called them 'sloths' and 'fidgets'. The sloths, between meals and toilet breaks, sat almost immobile, slumped in their easy chairs, reading or listening to the radio. The fidgets were almost never still – they shifted around in their chairs, drummed their fingers on the arm rests, often got up and walked around and spent time doing little jobs, such as writing or creating objects from materials left in the room, rather than sitting still.

The results were not as expected. The fidgets tended to lose weight or maintain their initial weight, while the sloths all gained weight, usually several pounds. That wasn't the surprise, as previous observations had persuaded the researchers that there did seem to be these two populations of people. The surprise was what the two groups had eaten.

Despite gaining weight, the sloths had actually eaten less than the fidgets. Most of the time, the fidgets had cleared their plates – they apparently had bigger appetites than the sloths. The conclusion had to be that the sloths gained weight not because they ate more, but because they exercised less.

I've been a doctor long enough to know that each generation seems to have forgotten the lessons of the previous one and the fidget and sloth study, reported in the early 1960s or perhaps even earlier, was certainly forgotten. It came as a surprise to the experts of the time, therefore (though not to me as the fidgets and sloths are ever present when I see obese patients), when an article on obesity in the European Union stated that there was half the rate of obesity among physically active people as there was among people who led sedentary lifestyles. M. A. Martinez-Gonzales, the lead author of the article (1999), wrote that a reduction in energy expenditure in leisure time may be the main determinant of the current epidemic of obesity.

Then came the bombshell from the USA's annual National Health and Nutrition Examination Survey (NHANES). It is a study that has been going on for decades into the general health of the American people. By 2003, it was reporting on the data gathered between 1971 and 1992. Its conclusion? The calorie intake of obese people was lower than that of thinner people. What was the main difference between these two groups of people? The heavier ones ate less but took far less exercise than the lighter ones. It wasn't the food they ate but the lack of exercise they took that was making them fat and, therefore, more than normally prone to heart attack, stroke, diabetes and even cancer.

By 2005, *The Lancet*, the internationally renowned British journal for doctors, was getting in on the sloths versus fidgets line. An article by S. Y. Kimm and colleagues following a study of teenage American girls clearly connected their exercise levels with their physiques, concluding that the more physically active they were, the less likely they were to be obese. The relationship was much stronger than any connection between what they ate and their shape or weight.

My memory of that 'sloths versus fidgets' lecture was being confirmed time and again by the facts. Crucial to our good health is that we are physically active. We are getting fatter as a population because we have stopped being physical and have become inert. The first lesson in getting thinner if we are overweight has to be to get physical. The second is that we don't necessarily lose weight by cutting down on our food intake – eating less if we don't exercise will hardly help us, if at all. If you want to lose weight simply by eating less because you have an aversion to exercise, then you will have to cut down the food you eat by such a great amount that you will always feel hungry or even starved – and you can't keep that up for the rest of your life.

So, could today's pandemic of obesity be simply or largely due to the fact that we are the first generation of human beings to move hardly at all? Is it true that sloths far outnumber fidgets, so today's social circumstances, where most physical jobs have become automated and we have become watchers of sport rather than participants in it, have made it so much easier to indulge our sloth tendencies?

Enter into the discussion Andy Coghlan of the *New Scientist* – my favourite writer in my favourite journal. On 29 August 2012, Andy wrote in the *New Scientist* about the 'workout pill'. He explained that it wasn't exactly a medication, but an exercise system, he has adopted. He escapes his office at 9 a.m. every morning to run up and down the fire escape for 20 minutes. By 2012, he had been doing it for eight years. The exercise 'pill' has brought down to normal his blood pressure, which was raised when he started the fire escape drill. He has 6 per cent less body fat than average for his age group and far less of it than average is to be found around his internal organs – a clear indication that he is at less risk than average of circulation problems such as heart attack and stroke. He can go longer on a treadmill than the average for his age and he has no known chronic illnesses. He asks his readers, if they were offered a pill that would do that for them, wouldn't they take it?

I confess, as one of his enthusiastic readers, I'm strongly on his side – and I do take his exercise 'pill'. I walk the hills near my home, I swim, I play golf (badly!) with like-minded mates on the rare Mondays when it doesn't rain in my beloved South West Scotland and I do a little destructive gardening a few days a week. I used to run half marathons, but I got to the stage and age that the organizers were sending out search parties for me because I couldn't keep up. So, I have gradually become less active in the last few years, which raises the question, 'How much do I still need to do to keep fit and healthy and avoid an expanding waistline?'

It's not easy to decide on an answer. There is a plethora of advice, not all based on properly conducted or analysed studies. For example, will a 40-minute walk each day do the trick or do we really need to get seriously out of breath four times a week? Should we exercise every day or is that bad for us? Is a hard workout just once a week enough, good or bad for us? Read any magazine or health column in a newspaper and you will find different answers to these questions. I confess that when I started to write this book, I was a bit confused myself, despite having handed out the same advice (get breathless three or four times a week) to my patients for decades.

Was what I was saying to them correct? Here is what I have managed to sift from the masses of advice on exercise in peer-reviewed journals and authorities on health, such as government bodies and universities. Andy Coghlan, for example, quotes the 'Exercise is Medicine' initiative by the American College of Sports Medicine, which has also collected together studies of people who have been following the US government's advice regarding how much physical activity to engage in. For you and me, that means two and a half hours a week of what is delightfully described as 'moderate intensity aerobic activity'. The College lists brisk walking, ballroom dancing and gardening in this category. Have you tried ballroom dancing for more than ten minutes? I have. It makes me more breathless than climbing a hill. You can try 75 minutes of what the College describes as 'more vigorous' activity, such as cycling, running and swimming instead.

Assuming that you are exercising five days a week, that is only 15 minutes a day of vigorous or half an hour of moderate exercise a day. It doesn't seem much in comparison with our hunter-gatherer ancestors' physical workload, yet the outcome is far beyond what we might expect. The Exercise is Medicine group showed that this relatively painless amount of weekly exercise reduced the numbers of premature deaths from heart disease by 40 per cent – curiously just the same fall as other studies have shown after the introduction of statin drugs prescribed to reduce cholesterol levels.

It appears that the benefit of exercise is universal. The Taiwan National Health Research Institute reported at the World Congress of Cardiology in April 2012 that exercise alone lowered the risk of heart attacks by between 30 and 50 per cent. The Taiwanese are thorough, including over 430,000 men and women in their study and following them for 12 years. Its leading author, Chi Pang Wen, explained that exercise works by widening the blood vessels, increasing the blood flow through them, and, in doing so, flushes out fats from their walls (quoted by Andy Coghlan, 2012). The effect is particularly important in the smaller arteries, in which narrowing leads to slowing of blood flow, the initial process that can lead to stroke.

The Chinese attitude to exercise has penetrated as far as our rural outpost in South West Scotland. For a few years now we have had a Xi Gong group in one of our villages. It started as a leisure activity for the retired, but our local medical practices, recognising the benefits reaped from it by these doughty pioneers, have started recommending it to their overweight and underfit middle- and older-aged patients.

Xi Gong is similar to Tai Chi (you will probably have seen the groups of Chinese elderly doing these exercises in city squares and parks) in that it involves slow and smooth exercises of all the muscles of the torso and limbs, repeated for up to an hour. It doesn't seem like you're exercising much to begin with, but, after 20 minutes of constant movement and challenges to your balance, you will change that opinion. Our sessions last for 45 minutes, then we are invited to lie down on a mat and rest completely for another 15. Never has 15 minutes of rest been more welcome! I was fairly fit when I started, but I am fitter now and I hate to miss a week. The group has expanded from around a dozen to the high twenties as people who are overweight, have diabetes, high blood pressure, heart problems and even anxiety states or depression have joined us. To a man and woman, we love it and I don't know of anyone whose medical condition hasn't improved as the weeks go by.

Of course, you don't need take my own anecdotal experience of obese patients who have responded to exercise by becoming fitter and healthier as the only evidence that it is vital. Read about the work of Steven Blair of the University of South Carolina. In 2009, his study of 50,000 men and women led him to conclude that lack of physical fitness (the sloths again, I'm afraid) was the cause of 16 per cent of all deaths. That is one person in six – greater than deaths from obesity, diabetes and high cholesterol added together! It is twice the numbers of deaths caused directly by smoking.

Christopher Hughes, Senior Lecturer at the University of London's Queen Mary Department of Sport and Exercise Medicine agrees with Dr Blair. In an interview with the *New Scientist*'s Andy Coghlan (2012), he emphasized that physical inactivity is a major killer. Dr Hughes told him that:

Everyone knows too much booze or tobacco is bad for you, but if physical inactivity was packaged and sold as a product, it would need to carry a health warning label.

How does exercise protect us from early death? One of its benefits is that it changes the types of fat circulated in your blood so that, in theory, it directly protects against catastrophic blocking of our arteries.

Everyone has heard of cholesterol, that it is a type of fat and if we have too much of it in our blood it can lead to heart attack and stroke. It seems that almost everyone over 50 years old has had a cholesterol test and many, if not most of us in that age group, are told its level in our blood is too high and we need to take statin drugs to reduce it. By doing so, we are told, we will halve our risk of an early (that is one occurring before we reach the age of 80) heart attack and stroke. That advice seems to be borne out by figures showing that since doctors started liberally dishing out statins to almost everyone approaching old age, the numbers of early deaths from these two major killers have fallen steeply.

The facts are not as simple as that, though. Rather than medicate half the population, wouldn't it be better to find another way to reduce the burden of such deaths? Does the evidence that exercise might do that stand up? Well, read the next few paragraphs, even though they are a bit technical.

First of all we *need* to transport fats around our body and we use cholesterol to do the logistics – look on it as the lorry carrying loads of different types of fats from the liver (where they are made from the fatty acids produced from digesting our food) to the tissues, then from the tissues back to the liver, where they are broken down into their basic components, ready for excretion. In normal living, a balance is struck between the two processes, with one type of fat – low-density lipoprotein (LDL) – being transported from the blood to the tissues and another – high-density lipoprotein (HDL) – removing the excess fat from the tissues and carrying it to the liver for excretion. There is a third type – very low-density lipoprotein (VLDL) or triglycerides – that performs the same job as LDL.

It is enough to state here that the higher the levels of LDL and VLDL or triglycerides in the blood, the more fatty 'streaks' we deposit on to the walls of our blood vessels. The higher our HDL, the better are our chances of removing these deposits so that they do not build up into the clumps of fat that are the initial sites of weakness and irregularities where bleeds into the walls and clots inside them can occur.

A problem arises when we have our cholesterol levels measured. We have all heard of 'high cholesterol' and we know of people who are being treated for it – to try to bring it down. The standard line is that if we have a cholesterol level above 5 millimoles per litre of blood (written as mmols/L), then we should do all we can to reduce it – preferably to below 4.5 mmol/L. However, the total cholesterol measurement doesn't take into account the relative values of LDL or triglycerides and HDL.

Take my levels as an example. My total cholesterol is 7.7 mmol/L, but HDL is a considerable component of that figure, at 2.3 mmol/L. That means my ratio of total cholesterol (TC) to HDL cholesterol is only 3.3 (7.7 divided by 2.3). That is important, because it is then well below 5, the point above which we know the risk of heart attack begins to rise. So, despite my having what people might think is a very high cholesterol level, I wouldn't do anything to disturb my very beneficial TC:HDL ratio. I don't take statins and my doctor agrees with that decision.

In 2012, Iqbal Al-Shayji, Muriel Caslake and Jason Gill and colleagues at the University of Glasgow reported that just two hours of exercise was enough to change the ratio of the fats in our blood in a way that protects us from the risk of stroke and heart attack. That amount of exercise caused blood levels of VLDL to fall by a quarter – a very significant protective effect. In many people, it would reduce the TC:HDL ratio to well below the crucial 5 level.

Of course, this was a research finding in an experiment conducted in a gymnasium linked to a laboratory, but how relevant is it to real life? The results from the Exercise is Medicine group strongly suggest that it is relevant. Among their subjects, people who exercised moderately just once a week were 58 per cent less at risk of becoming diabetic than people who didn't. As diabetes greatly increases our risk of heart attack and stroke, this would lead to many years of extra healthy life among those who, had they not taken up exercise, would have developed the disease. Remember the risk of diabetes for the Pima described in the previous chapter? The same story is echoed in those of their fellow Americans in the Exercise is Medicine study. There are plenty of case histories (among my own patients, too) of obese type 2 diabetics who, by exercising more, lose their disease along with their excess weight.

'Diabetes isn't all that common', I can almost hear you mutter to yourself. 'I don't have diabetes in my family, so it isn't a risk for me.' Please think again. Type 2 diabetes (the one that arises in adults and is linked to being overweight) *was* rare in the 1930s. According to Diabetes UK, the main organisation in the UK devoted to diabetes care and research, in the mid-1930s, when the total population worldwide was only 2 billion, around 15 million people had type 2 diabetes. We were thin then! By 2010, though, with 7 billion people on the earth, Diabetes UK reported that 220 million of them had type 2 diabetes. The world's population had trebled and the number of people with diabetes had multiplied 15 times over. We are not thin now. That reminds me of another of my 'connections' from the beginning of the Introduction.

In 1966, England won the Football (Soccer for American readers) World Cup. Scotland didn't do so well, so when the Scottish team beat England at Wembley in 1967, you can imagine, given the rivalry between the two countries, that the Scots supporters ran wild. Unfortunately, they invaded the pitch, climbing on to the goal cross bar and breaking it. They also took a few squares of Wembley turf home with them, presumably to supplement their lawns. To give them their due, the Scots paid for all the repairs, but there remains on film the antics of that famous (if you are Scottish) or notorious (if you are English) day.

What intrigues me now about that film is there isn't a single fat fan in the whole scene. Everyone is slim and fit-looking – and apparently very physically active, judging from their ability to run from and avoid the stewards and police by 'jinking and jiving', as the Scottish call it! If there were any obese diabetic fans there, they were absolutely not visible.

Less than 40 years later, the fans were very different. I chose the film of the England v. Sweden match in 2005 to use for comparison, but it could be any football match in the English league today. There is hardly a slim fan to be seen. The spectators are seated, so forced to be less active than the standing fans of 1967, but that doesn't explain their different physiques. I accept, of course, that it was right from a safety point of view to make seating compulsory at football grounds after the well-known tragedies caused by crushing injuries among the standing fans pushed in waves against barriers and fences, but the now less active (sitting for an hour and three quarters is much less energetic than standing for the same time) fans are, almost all, overweight. It is hard to believe that such a massive change could have occurred in such a short time.

Katherine Flegal, Margaret Carroll, Brian Kit and Cynthia Ogden (2012) reported in the *Journal of the American Medical Association* (JAMA) that a third of American men and women are obese. Worse still, Ogden, Carroll, Kit and Flegal (2012) found that one in six American children is obese. Remember that the definition of obesity is much more severe than simply being overweight. People who are classified as obese are so overweight that they are definitely at harm from their excess. In the USA, that means at least 20 per cent above the normal weight for their height. So, these figures don't even begin to reflect the true scale of the problem – the many millions more who are overweight, but not included in the obesity statistics.

Linked to obesity, along with diabetes, come early death and disability. The USA is the richest nation in the world, but it is by no means the healthiest, nor are Americans the longest-lived people. In December 2012, *The Lancet* devoted a whole issue to the results of the 'Global Burden of Disease Study' (GBD). This is serious stuff. GBD is the first comprehensive survey of disease and health risks since 1990. It is the result of the combined efforts of seven institutions: Harvard University, the University of Washington in Seattle, Johns Hopkins University, the University of Queensland, Imperial College, London, the University of Tokyo and the World Health Organisation (WHO). It is supported by the Bill and Melinda Gates Foundation.

It lists and ranks every country for its life expectancy and its 'healthy life expectancy'. So many more people are living longer than in the past, but enduring years of poor health before they die, that the two figures can diverge widely. It makes interesting reading. At the top of the lists for men and women (they are calculated separately) are Japan, Singapore, Switzerland and Spain. South Korean women are healthier than their menfolk and Italian men do better than their wives, but both sexes in both countries do far better than their counterparts in the USA. The Greeks are well up the healthy living list, too. US males, though, come 32nd and females 35th on the list for healthy life expectancy, 12 and 6 places behind their equivalents in the UK. Some of that difference comes from lives lost due to violence, but the main difference in health between the USA and the countries above it is its high rate of obesity and especially type 2 diabetes.

It is no coincidence that Japanese, South Koreans and Singaporeans live healthily for so much longer than the Brits and the Americans. As nations, they are far slimmer and have traditions of more physical activity in their daily lives than Westerners. Switzerland's highly healthy population isn't put down to its obvious material wealth, but to its tradition, too, of physical activity, such as skiing and hill walking – although even Switzerland, traditionally slimmer than Germany, has been getting fatter in recent years. This is largely due to its people partaking in less physical activity and, sadly, the trend starts young – for example, children being driven to school instead of walking.

What about the Spanish, Italians and Greeks? Until relatively recently, anyone going to the countries around the Mediterranean might well have been impressed by how slim the people still were. With their traditional Mediterranean diet, its emphasis on olive oil, fresh and local produce and fish and habit of slow-paced, family meals, their eating habits compared very favourably with those of the UK. Even now, many still adhere to this, especially in rural areas where the traditional way of life is still maintained, with plenty of physical activity. They eat exceptionally well, sensibly, slowly and never too much. They drink their wine with their meals and make them the social event of their day.

Sadly, however, as the Mediterranean diet has declined, so obesity has risen. It's a growing problem in Spain as eating habits have changed and people are abandoning the traditional diet in favour of high-fat and high-sugar snacks. Lack of exercise is also to blame. Statistics suggest that some 40 per cent of Spanish youths never practise sport and are becoming lazier and heavier, with increasing exposure to the Internet and video games, as well as television. According to a 2012 report by the Organisation for Economic Co-operation and Development (OECD), 30 per cent of its teenagers are overweight, putting Spain just behind America and Scotland for obesity. The OECD also predicts that the number of overweight people will rise by a further 10 per cent over the next decade. The Spanish health ministry already spends 2.5 billion euros a year on obesity-related illnesses. Two out of three men are already overweight in Spain, while one in six people is obese.

The story is even worse in Italy, where 36 per cent of Italian children are overweight or obese by the age of eight, according to a survey by the Institute for Auxology of Milan (Archenti and Pasqualinotto, 2008). It's a similar story – people are forgetting the traditional way of eating in favour of fast foods, with the result that 10 per cent of the adult Italian population is officially obese and 35 per cent overweight.

In Greece, two thirds of children and three quarters of adults are overweight and a United Nations report said the diet in western Crete, considered the birthplace of the Mediterranean diet, had 'decayed into a moribund state'.

It's a very clear, if frightening, demonstration in our lifetime (almost as we watch) of what happens when people suddenly switch from the diet that has served them so well for centuries and start consuming the Western diet at its worst – high in refined flours, sugars and fats. As we know to our cost, it's a diet that fuels a future of diseases such as cardiovascular disease, diabetes and cancer.

The most spectacular of these diseases, and most discussed in the media, has been diabetes, linked as it has been to early deaths from various causes. Its 15-fold rise in the developed world is not only directly related to obesity but also a direct cause of the lowly position of the USA – and, to some extent, the UK – on the ladder of healthy life expectancy. That alone is more than enough reason to take up exercise. There are many more proven benefits of exercise, however, some of which may surprise you. How much have you heard, for example, of the benefits of exercise in preventing cancer?

Let's turn back again to the Exercise is Medicine initiative (mentioned on page 16). The College found that when people followed the US government's advice on exercise – moderate exercise for

two and a half hours or vigorous exercise for 75 minutes a week –
women lowered their risk of breast cancer by half and men and
women lowered their risk of bowel cancer by 60 per cent. This is
huge protection, exceeding anything that a medicine or any other
lifestyle change has ever been shown to produce. A small dose of
aspirin (75 mg a day) approaches the effect on bowel cancer, but
the evidence for a similar effect to that of aspirin on breast cancer
is equivocal.

How does exercise do this? It may be simply that if you start exercising you lose weight. Excess weight is linked to breast cancer in
postmenopausal women, so, if they exercise it away, their chances
of avoiding cancer increase steeply. There may be more to it than
that, however. If you are carrying extra fat in your storage tissues
(around your waist and your internal organs) your blood carries
around it higher levels of substances that researchers have found
to promote cancer. They include female hormones, growth factors
and chemicals that promote inflammation. Losing the fat reduces
the levels of these substances in the blood and the effect of this is
greater the more fat you lose.

What is true of breast cancer studies is even more emphatic for
bowel cancer. Dr Anne McTiernan, a cancer prevention researcher
at the Fred Hutchinson Cancer Research Center in Seattle, has
managed to persuade 200 healthy subjects to undergo bowel biopsies and was able to divide them into 'exercisers' and 'non-exer-
cisers'. Having worked in medical research for seven years, most
of which time was spent trying to set up clinical trials with volunteers, I fully understand how difficult that must have been. She
then had to examine each of the biopsies microscopically to be able
to predict which of the specimens might be prone to later developing cancer. The clue was in the 'crypts' in the bowel wall. These are
deep folds in the surface, like crevasses in a glacier, that are essential for absorption of water and the uptake of nutrients through
the bowel wall. They provide a wide surface area for good contact
between the bowel contents and the inside surface of the gut.

Dr McTiernan found that cells in the crypts of her 'sloths' were
far more actively dividing than those in the crypts of the 'fidgets'.
It is the more actively dividing cells that are more likely to form
fleshy masses such as polyps, which are often the precursors

of cancer. Why exercise should have this effect on the bowel is unknown, but it is significant and was a constant finding in Dr McTiernan's studies (reported at a conference on aspirin in cancer in November 2012).

Is exercise turning out to be the modern equivalent of the panacea, the universal health-giving, disease-curing medicine that ancient doctors sought since the days of Hippocrates around 300 BC? So far we have heard that it helps people to keep healthier longer and live longer, how it prevents the onset of, and even reverses established, diabetes. There is strong evidence that it prevents cancers of the breast and bowel (and perhaps prostate, too) and it generally makes you feel and function better. Are we going too far, suggesting that it is a panacea?

Well, here is another thought. Would you believe that regular exercise may prevent dementia? In 2011 my publishers, Sheldon Press, asked me to write a book on what we can do to prevent us from developing dementia. Like many other doctors, I began the research for the book believing there wasn't much we could do for ourselves on that score, except to avoid the obvious promoters of brain deterioration, such as excess alcohol, smoking, professional boxing and other dangerous sports that can put you at risk of head injuries.

How wrong I was. As I delved into the literature, I discovered that being physically active is vital to protect and even develop the brain. The most effective brain protector is to learn a musical instrument when young and, if you are good enough, to play regularly in a professional orchestra. Professional classical musicians are surprisingly resistant to Alzheimer's type dementia. It is thought the protection comes from a combination of characteristics, one being that to play an instrument to a high standard involves many hours of practice, using all your senses. It is not simply a matter of manual dexterity, but immense coordination of all the senses, of hearing, touch, learning the new oral and complex written language of musical scores and, most of all, perhaps, working happily with your fellow musicians. Members of orchestras are famously gregarious and enjoy a good social life. Next time you go to a concert, try to spot a fat musician. They are as rare as hen's teeth – or a fat boy in my old school photograph.

One example, however, is not enough. It may be that people who become musicians are genetically programmed to avoid dementia or the ones who will develop dementia never quite make it past the auditions for the top orchestras. Interestingly, neither explanation holds water. It turns out that if you start a new interest such as learning to play an instrument even when you are older, you can put the dementia prevention process in place for your own brain. That is, provided you do so in the company of other like-minded enthusiasts – it is no good being solitary.

Up to, say, ten years ago, I wouldn't have believed exercise could have this effect on the brain. We were taught in medical school that our brains developed until we were in our late teenage years or early twenties, then deteriorated at a regular rate thereafter. We started, so went the dogma, to lose brain nerve cells (our neurones) by the million every few days (don't worry, there are plenty to lose) so that by the time we were in our seventies, we were scratching around to get a few to work together. That's a bit of an exaggeration, but we believed that this was a fundamental part of being human and the ageing process.

Now, though, we know that we can replace old brain cells and even make new ones. We can open up pathways between the two halves of our brains and use them to keep ourselves bright and intelligent. One of the keys to the research that arrived at this very encouraging conclusion came from studies of London cabdrivers in the 1970s. UK readers will remember that London cabbies have been prominent in the *Brain of Britain* on BBC Radio and *Mastermind* television programme contests since they started. Why should cabbies be such brainboxes?

London is unique in that the black cab drivers must learn and pass an examination in 'The Knowledge' before being given a licence to carry passengers. Look at a map of London's streets and imagine how you might memorize them. Would-be cabbies have to do exactly that. Some do so by driving around the streets, remembering landmarks such as pubs and churches, others do it by poring over the maps for hours on end. However they manage it, by the time they have finished the task, they have laid down a mass of new nerve pathways and nerve cells in their brains. Crucial to this are two areas of the brain – the corpus callosum, which is the 'bridge' between the two halves of the brain, and the hippocampus, an area deep within the brain that is thought to coordinate memories and reasoning. Apparently, learning The Knowledge enhances both of these areas (Woollett and Maguire, 2011) and, in doing so, it gives them an extra capacity for other intellectual pursuits.

What has this got to do with exercise? I hope they will forgive me for writing this, but London cabbies aren't well known for exercising. Since the original studies of their brains pointed to a way of measuring improvements and changes in the brain and its activity, however, scans have been used to look at many other groups of people undergoing intellectual tests. You have guessed what is coming next. If you exercise, you will stimulate your brain, too, in precisely the same areas that cabbies use to learn The Knowledge.

So, in a way, exercise does indeed go a long way towards being the panacea that, you will recall, the doctors of long ago were searching for. Again, don't take my word for it, try to find *The Lancet* of 21 July 2012. On the front cover is emblazoned the statement:

> Worldwide, we estimated that physical inactivity causes 6–10% of the major non-communicable diseases . . . physical inactivity seems to have an effect similar to that of smoking or obesity.

Inside there is a 58-page section devoted to how the whole world's population's levels of physical activity have changed, usually for the worse, and how that has affected our health. It is heavy reading, but it is important, as the messages in it are serious, to say the least, so I'll try to tease out the key points and make them readable.

The data for adults came from 122 countries and for adolescents (defined as 13- to 15-year-olds) from 105, so are very wide-ranging. The raw facts are that 31 per cent of all adults are physically inactive, but that covers a wide range. For example you would probably guess that people are more active in poorer countries than in richer ones, so that only 4.7 per cent of Bangladeshis (both men and women) are inactive will not surprise you. What about the figure of 71.9 per cent for Malta, though?

Europe as a whole has still to catch up with North America in the sloth stakes: 43 per cent of Americans, but only 34 per cent of Europeans, are classified as physically inactive. Much worse for the future, 80 per cent of all 13- to 15-year-olds are active for under an hour a day, boys being more active than girls.

These figures mean that a third of adults and four-fifths of teenagers in the developed countries do not reach public health guidelines for recommended levels of physical activity. In other words, among the young, sloths far outnumber fidgets.

How do *The Lancet's* authors define 'physical inactivity'? Measuring physical activity became extremely technical from the late 1990s onwards. Trust academics to come up with a precise way of measuring it. They first devised the International Physical Activity Questionnaire (IPAQ), testing its validity and reliability in 12 countries before developing it into the Global Physical Activity Questionnaire (GPAQ), then asking all the countries participating in the survey to use it. The data so far collected using this questionnaire and reported in 2012 have come from two thirds of all countries and represent 88.9 per cent of the world population. It is difficult to argue with such numbers.

So, are you physically inactive according to the parameters? Do you measure up or not? Here is where I get a little technical again. Don't worry, it is fairly straightforward.

You are classified as physically inactive if you do not meet any of the following three criteria:

- you do not undergo 30 minutes of moderate intensity activity on at least 5 days a week
- or 20 minutes of vigorous physical activity on at least 3 days a week
- or a combination of the two that amounts to 600 metabolic equivalent minutes (MET) a week.

One MET is the energy we expend when we are sitting quietly. Multiply that by 8 for every minute you exercise vigorously or 4 for moderate activity, such as walking. So, if you run for 30 minutes 3 days a week, that is 3 x 240 = 720 MET – well above the upper level set as defining you as inactive. When measuring activity, of course, all aspects of your life have to be included, such as time spent doing housework or walking or cycling to work – it is not just activity in our leisure time that is taken into account. When all this is factored into the calculations, it takes very little exercise, really, to achieve the exalted status of being a physically active person. The converse is, of course, that someone labelled as physically inactive is hardly moving at all!

Take walking, for example. Almost exactly two-thirds of us, men and women, regardless of the country in which we live, walk for at least ten minutes at a time on at least five days a week. That is a good start (200 points) towards fulfilling our MET quota, but it isn't enough on its own. When it comes to more vigorous activity, only around a third of us take part in it on three or more days a week. That figure drops to a quarter in North America and Europe, with the most active people living in South East Asia (43 per cent) and in the Western Pacific (35 per cent). It is probably not a coincidence that this is where people live longest and keep healthiest until their old age.

Crucial to interpreting these results is what the authors call 'active transportation' or commuting to work by foot or bicycle. A host of studies have reported that people who get to and from work by using their legs live longer and have fewer illnesses than people who use cars, trains or buses. This is particularly important for schoolchildren. Boys and girls who walk or cycle to and from school weigh less and have better cardiovascular fitness than those whose parents take them by car.

Comparisons made between countries make stark reading. Fewer than 2 per cent of people in Australia, Canada, Ireland, the UK and the USA cycle to work or school. More than 20 per cent do so in China (which is not surprising, I suppose), Denmark and the Netherlands. Of course, the provision of dedicated cycle lanes matters a lot in the decision to cycle. The Dutch have always had them and the Danes have seen a 50 per cent increase in cycling since they followed the Netherlands' example and instituted them from the 1990s onwards.

The Danes have even estimated from their results that if all non-cyclists started pedalling, they would prevent 12,000 deaths a year that are currently attributed to lack of physical activity and only lose 30 cyclists in the same time from traffic accidents. The fact that there are many more cyclist deaths in countries with less cycle-friendly roads stops most of us from following the Dutch and Danes. On the basis of the Danish experience, if we could make cycling to school and work easier and safer, we would save tens of thousands of lives and keep many more people healthier into our sixties and seventies. Why don't we go ahead and do it? In the long run, we would save millions in medicines and care costs, but, most of all, we would have a much healthier older population.

We have to start people on this course young. Here is another acronym for you – HBSC, which stands for 'Health behaviour in school-aged children', the World Health Organization's (WHO) ongoing survey of children in 43 European and North American countries and regions, conducted and a report produced every four years. It showed (*The Lancet*, 2012) that two thirds of boys (66 per cent) and a few more girls (68 per cent) spend more than two hours a day watching television. More than a third of them sit for more than three hours a day. Other WHO studies report that around half of all adults now spend more than four hours of their waking day sitting around doing nothing physical and the periods of time we do so get longer as we grow older.

Do these figures really matter? The Danes certainly think so and, on the basis of all the evidence that has been accruing on our general slothdom, everyone else should support them, but can we change things?

First, we need to know why we modern humans really don't seem to like exercise and physical activity when we have, as a species, been programmed to be active for millions of years. It is only in the last generation that our habits have changed. I have devoted the next chapter to that subject, but let me return to the cruise I mentioned in Chapter 2 for a moment and my last conversation with the ship's doctor.

You will recall that the cruise took the form of boarding at Los Angeles, travelling for five days on the ocean to Hawaii, five days visiting the various islands and five days sailing back to Los Angeles. On the morning after we had finally left the islands, the young woman with anorexia was not in the pool. In fact, she didn't appear again. I was curious, but knew enough about medical etiquette not to pry. On the last evening, my doctor friend opened up to me. He had had a hard decision to make while at the last port of call. Could he risk allowing her to travel for five days without the possibility of fast access to specialist care when she was showing signs that she might go into heart failure?

She had fainted in her cabin shortly after one of her swimming sessions and, on being called to see her by her mother, he had found that her heart was beating irregularly. She weighed 6 stone, 6 lbs (41 kilograms, 90 lbs), which for a woman of around 5 feet 6 inches (1.67 m) tall was seriously below normal. It wasn't easy for him. She was facing five days at sea, for three of which she would be well out of range if she needed to be rescued by helicopter. The cruise company could not risk the consequences if she died suddenly, especially as the possibility had been raised before leaving Hawaii. Neither she nor her mother had wanted to leave the ship, but he was firm. He arranged for her to fly home to California and be admitted to a heart unit there.

So, not all exercise is good. We mustn't overdo it, especially if we are already underweight. Overexercising when we are not replacing the energy we expend is disastrous: we soon lose our fat stores, then we lose muscle. When our bodies start to use up heart muscle for energy, we are in deep trouble and, sadly, the young woman with anorexia would not accept that this was precisely what was happening to her. Sudden heart failure is often the cause of death among anorexics. It is such a shame that it is so difficult to help them through this very serious illness.

One last comment on exercise and obesity. The Fukushima Nuclear Power Station disaster in Japan was a tragedy that saddened the world. Among all the fears for the health of the population in and around the contaminated area, one unexpected consequence has emerged (*Japan Times*, 2012). There are still restrictions on outdoor activities for children at the local primary schools nearest to the Fukushima site, so the pupils are less physically active than they were. Within two years, they were significantly heavier for their height than they had been before the tragedy and they were fatter, too, than the children in similar schools outside the Fukushima region, where there are no restrictions on outdoor activities. The schools in both regions provide the same food and, apart from the ban on outdoor activities, the two groups of children have exactly the same lifestyles. The only reason for their extra weight, therefore, appears to be that they are exercising less than they should. It is sad proof of the relationship between exercise and weight that the Japanese would rather they had never had to discover in this way.

That brings us to the subject of obesity in children.

Overweight and obese children

Many mothers have to be told that their children are becoming overweight. They do not always recognize it themselves, as the researchers using ScotCen Social Research Group's 'Growing Up in Scotland' study data found and note in their report (Parkes, Sweeting and Wight, 2012).

The researchers examined data concerning the health of almost 3000 children and their parents, with a particular emphasis on weight. Sadly, Scotland has one of the highest levels of child obesity in the Western world, with 22 per cent of Scottish six-year-olds being overweight and 9 per cent classified as obese. So, the report was timely and Scotland is an appropriate country from which the rest of the UK could learn.

From these figures you can calculate that one in five of the children in the study was overweight, yet hardly any mothers recognized that fact. Of the children who were already overweight or obese by the time they were six years old, only one in seven of their mothers was concerned. Asked to classify their children from four categories – very overweight, somewhat overweight, normal weight or underweight – 86 per cent of the mothers of obese or overweight children described them as of normal weight.

Strangely, the vast majority of overweight and obese mothers put themselves in the correct category when asked to do so and were usually concerned about their own health, yet they did not see the same pattern in their children. I have a personal memory of this, when, years ago, I tried gently to tell a mother that her daughter was obese and needed to adopt a new lifestyle. There was a bucket of soapy water on the floor beside her that she had been using to wash her windows. It was upturned over my head, because I had dared to criticize her perfect daughter. Tragically, the family then left the practice because of my perceived rudeness. I heard years later that the poor girl had died in her early thirties in her sleep. By that time she had become morbidly obese and had simply stopped breathing in the night – 'sleep apnoea' is a common way for the morbidly obese to die.

'Growing Up in Scotland' found that mothers were less likely to recognize weight problems in their sons than in their daughters. Fathers did not seem to come into the discussion at all – obesity in the children seemed to be linked, if anything, to the mother's rather than the father's weight. A surprising conclusion was that hours spent in front of the television did not seem to influence a child's weight. Apart from an overweight or obese mother, the major influences that led to a child being overweight or obese included eating sweets and crisps as a toddler, skipping breakfast, not eating an evening meal at the family dining table and low levels of parental supervision.

The very clear message from the report is that childhood obesity is a result of poor family interactions and the failure of parents even to recognize it. The answer, therefore, is not to concentrate on the child, but on relationships within the family and its overall lifestyle. Children have to be active, but their parents must be, too. The secret is for the parents to spend more time engaged in active physical effort with their children and for the whole family to find some hobbies or sports that they can all enjoy together. It is a simple message, but one that requires a lot of effort from parents and children alike.

The alternative is not an option. It is not enough for a mother to be persuaded to recognize that her child is overweight. The survey found that even when children were correctly identified as being overweight at the age of four, they were still overweight or had even progressed to being obese two years later. Parents must take up the challenge to reverse the trend as early as possible and that takes a lot of effort from them.

They may derive some help from the results of the National Child Measurement Programme, now running in every primary school in England. If a mother or father is doubtful about the weight status of their child, the Programme provides an objective, unbiased assessment that can hardly be disputed. Schools are also much more aware of the need for physical activity and are, thankfully, less willing than they were to excuse obese children from games and physical education. They may also be more used than doctors to having buckets of water thrown over them! Joking aside, the prime mover in preventing or reversing a child being overweight is his or her parents. Mothers and fathers have no excuse now that they have so many people on their children's side to help them.

3

Why we don't exercise enough

If becoming physically active is so good for us, why do so many of us not want to exert ourselves? Why do we prefer to be couch potatoes? Are we genetically programmed to be lazy and dislike being active or is it something we learn or are forced into by our environment? If so, can we unlearn our dislike and find it as enjoyable as we surely did as children? You won't be surprised to know that there has been plenty of research into all of this and you will be even less surprised, perhaps, to learn that it has produced few hard and fast conclusions.

The best review of the causes of our general dislike of exercise – entitled 'Correlates of physical activity: Why are some people physically active and others not? – appeared in *The Lancet* (Bauman, Reis, Sallis, Wells, Loos and Martin, 2012), produced for the Lancet Physical Activity Series Working Group. I love its approach: it divides the aspects of life that determine physical activity into:

- sleep
- leisure time
- occupation
- transportation
- home-based activities

or SLOTH! I wonder how long it took for them to devise that acronym, but it is about as appropriate as acronyms can be. SLOTH becomes immediately useful when looking at its five aspects in relation to different social classes and countries. For example, until recently, the occupation, home-based and transportation divisions were important for determining levels of physical activity in low- and middle-income countries and populations and leisure time was the most active aspect of SLOTH for richer countries and people. The division between the haves and have nots has lessened in recent years as industrialization has reached the poorer and more rural countries and their people have begun to abandon walking and cycling in favour of buses, trains and cars.

China is a good example. A. C. Bell, K. Ge and B. M. Popkin (2002) summed up the situation in the title of their article: 'The road to obesity or the path to prevention: Motorized transportation and obesity in China'. They reported on the massive increase in body mass index (a reliable marker for obesity) in China that is directly related to the transition from cycling to car use in adults. The numbers of motor vehicles multiplied ten-fold in China between 1990 and 2005. The lesson of the Pima will have to be learned again in China and in every developing country that is adopting a motorized economy.

Some countries are tackling the problem with more vigour, and better results, than others. The best example is in Bogotá, capital of Colombia. There, a forward-looking government has recognized the need to keep its citizens healthy and happy while undergoing the transition to becoming a modern society. Understanding that universal access to easy, effective and affordable transport was the key, the authorities instituted two mutually and highly compatible systems – the TransMilenio bus rapid transport system (BRT) and the Ciclovia, which is the closing, at least once a week, of streets in the city to allow people to be as physically active in as many ways as they wish.

The BRT buses run in exclusive lanes, have well-planned routes and stops and carry 1.4 million passengers every day. They are the fastest and most efficient way of moving around the city and studies have already shown that the BRT has encouraged Bogotáns of all classes to be more active physically – simply by walking to and from the buses and making the most of the opportunities that the bus service has opened up to them.

The Ciclovia also adds hugely to the citizens' opportunities to keep active and happy. During the Ciclovia, which takes place every Sunday and on numerous holidays too, around 60 miles (97 km) of the city's streets are closed for 7 hours at a time. They are turned over to pedestrians, rollerbladers, runners and cyclists. It involves input from the departments of education, health, sports, culture and recreation, transport, the police, urban planning and local government. It appears to run smoothly and costs the city about US $1.7 million a year, but is well worth the trouble, time and effort. The latest estimates suggest that the value of the benefits in health and prevention of illness among Bogotáns since Ciclovia was established has outweighed its costs by approximately four-fold.

Some 90 per cent of the people taking part in Ciclovia are from the poorer sections of Bogotán society, so if it were not available to them, many would be so sedentary that they would be classed as 'physically inactive' according to the WHO's categories described in the previous chapter. Now the people meet the physical activity recommendations for good health. Many of them cycle regularly and admit that they would not be doing so if the Ciclovia had not been there for them.

Since Bogotá took the lead, Ciclovias have been established in more than 100 other Latin American cities. They have been hugely popular with the people, who view them as their main source of enjoyment in life. Some 17 of the 35 countries in the Americas now promote Ciclovias and the early signs are that they have already produced significant improvements in the health of their people.

That seems to be the key – enjoyment of life. The Ciclovias provide exercise that is in the right form, in the right environment, among like-minded companions, without costing the people anything and providing them with the right motivation. People don't go to the Ciclovias because they 'want to lose weight' or even 'to keep healthy' or to 'prevent future illness', they go because they enjoy them. They give them a mixture of fun, opportunities to meet with friends and feel good by being physically active all at the same time. They aren't in a gym or taking part in organized workout sessions or paying fees and no one is preaching the health message at them. They simply love the feeling of being social human beings together with many others who feel the same way.

If the Bogotáns have managed to be so successful in reversing the Pima-like trend towards a population that was simply becoming fatter and fatter, can the rest of the world follow their example?

Must we provide free transport, traffic-free streets and lay on all sorts of entertainment to do so? Maybe it is more difficult in the much wealthier and more money orientated societies of Europe and North America, but that's not a reason to ignore this positive evidence from Latin America.

To explore this, let's return to the Lancet Physical Activity Series Working Group mentioned above. Its research showed that, above all other personal factors, confidence in our ability to be physically active is vital. A poor self-image tends to make us look inwards, mentally and physically, so that we move towards the inert, rather than the energetic. If, along with lack of confidence, we are over-weight, we are less likely to heed – in fact, we will positively reject – the message that we should become active. The sexes differ, too, with men being more likely to be active than women – a differ-ence that increases with age. Indeed, men and women perceive age almost as an excuse for becoming less active physically, which partially explains why both sexes accept middle-age spread – our expanding waistlines – as a normal part of ageing. It is common, yes, but not 'normal'. There is no physiological reason, other than underactivity (or, if you prefer, slothdom), for us to gain weight as we grow older.

That still doesn't answer the question, why would some of us rather not exercise if we can avoid it? It may be because some of us inherit a genetic make-up that makes us less physically active than others. That isn't fanciful. Studies of identical and non-identical twins and siblings in families strongly suggest there is an inherited component that appears to make us actively enjoy or dislike exer-cise. Indeed, in one study (Frayling, 2012) of more than 20,000 young adult twin pairs from eight European countries, the identi-cal twins were much closer to each other's body mass indices than the non-identical twins of the same sex – a clear indication that inheritance has something to do with the development of obesity (or, for that matter, thinness). A British study (Frayling, 2012) of 5000 twin pairs came to a similar conclusion. Both estimated that inheritance was around 70 per cent responsible for body shape (Frayling, 2012).

Dr E. J. de Geus and colleagues wrote about this and molecular aspects of sports performance in 2011. They divided people into those who have above average physical skills, who actually crave action and feel rewarded by accomplishing skilled athletic tasks, and those who feel pain or discomfort and easily become tired on slight or moderate exertion. They uncovered evidence that physical activity has links to the genetics underlying the brain's reward systems and sensation of pain. For some, the inherited balance when we exert ourselves is towards a sensation of reward, while for others it is towards one of pain. The critical genes that presumably determine the difference in responses have not yet been identified, however. Until they are we won't be able to understand fully why some of us really dislike any form of physical activity. That is a shame, because it makes it difficult for people who feel like this to manage to control their excess weight. If they don't begin to change their feelings about, and responses to, physical activity, they will never become active enough to lose their excess weight, so will continue to put it on instead.

If this is you, you will surely recognize the following. At the simplest level, you would rather lie in bed for a few minutes longer than take a walk in the fresh air round the garden before breakfast. You know you should take the stairs rather than the lift or escalator, but you can't be bothered. You tried to walk to the next bus stop rather than your nearest one for your commute to and from work, but you stopped it after a few days because it seemed pointless. You even joined a gym and meant to go once or twice a week, but quickly became bored and gave up your membership. Swimming was helpful for a week or two, but you decided that what seemed like endless pointless lengths up and down the pool were driving you mad – along with, it seemed, the rest of the swimmers who constantly bumped into you.

You have now concluded that exercising your fat away isn't for you and you lapse back into your old habits of near inertia. You begin to accept that you are one of those people who is genetically programmed to feel discomfort, or at the least unenthusiastic, when you exert yourself. You think it is unfortunate and that you can't change your inheritance, so you must live with it.

Wrong. There are ways to change. The best would be to take part in a Ciclovia, but that is probably too far for you to go if you don't live in Latin America. Its principles still apply, however. The first of these is that however you become active you must enjoy it – it must become one of the most enjoyable aspects of your life. Gyms, pools and exercise classes probably won't provide that.

How, then, do you turn yourself around from being, let's face it, someone who is a sloth and become a fidget instead? You can do it, but it is very difficult if you try to change by yourself. You need encouragement and, usually, the company of someone else in the same boat. That encouragement is vital, because most overweight people are both self-conscious and self-deprecating, lacking the one characteristic essential for success – self-confidence. You need others to help you build it up, which means family and friends supporting your change of lifestyle. If they are sloths, too, they must change with you: it is almost impossible to keep up the good work, even if you have started with enthusiasm, if you are sur-rounded by people who continue to remain inactive. Inveterate couch potatoes often hide from, or cope with, their own lack of drive by deriding the efforts of others and it is difficult to fight against them.

Slimming organizations

So, rule one is to recognize that you need to regain your self-con-fidence and, if friends and family aren't helping, then do so in the company of others. This is where organizations such as Slim-ming World and WeightWatchers have done so well. I have been impressed by their long-term results for some of their clients, not because of the diets they often promote, but because they base their improvements on exercise programmes with which their clients are comfortable and they can enjoy with others, who often become their close friends.

I admit that I was sceptical to begin with. All the evidence I had read suggested to me that their programmes work while the participants are still keen, but the enthusiasm usually wears off after around a year and between 80 and 90 per cent of them pile their weight on again to become fatter than ever. WeightWatchers' strength is that it has many years of experience in working with NHS Trusts in the UK to run weight loss programmes for people whose weight has put them at significant risk of serious illness.

Zoe Hellman, its head of dietetics and health policy, claims that the WeightWatchers programmes produce better results than their competitors and I'm happy to accept that. I'm just still a little dubious about any programme that involves calorie-counting restrictive diets.

The best independent evidence that I could find for the Weight-Watchers system was from S. Heshka and colleagues in 2003 in the *Journal of the American Medical Association*. The report looked at the results for 423 overweight and obese people who lost an average of just under 10 lbs (which is a bit less than 1 stone or 4.3 kg) in the first year. That was pretty impressive, as there must have been many who lost more to compensate for those who did not lose at all. A year later, however, the average loss compared to the start of their programme was only a little over 6 lbs (2.9 kg), indicating that they had put on 3lbs (1.4 kg) in their second 12-month period.

The Slimming World system does not involve the use of the word 'diet'. The aim is healthy eating, which means lots of fruit, salads, vegetables, lean meat, fish, cheese, pasta, rice and pulses. Nothing is left out and, according to the representative I interviewed for this book, there is no calorie counting. At least as important as eating well for Slimming World clients is exercise. Newcomers to the group start off slowly and increase their exercises week by week, and they enjoy it. It is called 'body magic' and may well be to some of the newcomers who have not exercised for a long time.

According to Lisa Boucher, the Slimming World consultant I interviewed, of her total of 350 members, 76 had reached their target weight, 50 of whom were still attending every week. The others were content to carry on by themselves, but Lisa was still in touch with them, making regular friendly phone calls.

The first six weeks, Lisa told me, are critical. During this time she guides all her group through their exercises each week and keeps a close eye on the newcomers. She texts her members every week to keep them enthusiastic – most of them go through sticky patches from time to time and Lisa feels responsible for guiding them through these.

There can be problems. Far more women than men join: only 12 out of her 350 current slimmers are men. She would like to have more, but the popular image of slimmers is almost entirely of women. Yet the men take to Slimming World more easily, they reach their target weights sooner and are more likely to stay at them afterwards.

Some slimmers can't stop. Lisa is acutely aware that they can go too far. If they reach a BMI of 20 or below, she has to expel them! She knows of the dangers of initiating anorexia, as well as of failure to help people lose weight.

I'm sure the WeightWatchers system trains its consultants as professionally as does Slimming World and that it works as well. They do seem to offer an ideal way to lose your excess weight if you are the sort of person who needs support when doing so – which means most of us. Both systems combine exercise with eating healthily: one watches calories and the other doesn't, so you can choose which system suits you better. The real bonus for either set of clients, however, lies in the pleasure of regularly meeting up with friends who are like-minded. Their support and the self-belief that they induce are essential for long-term success. I am happy to refer patients to either organization.

Overeaters Anonymous (<www.oagb.org.uk/>) is a 12-step fellowship of people who view obesity as just one of many symptoms or manifestations of an underlying urge towards compulsive eating. Accordingly, meetings focus on emotional and spiritual components involved in eating, rather than actual weight loss and gain, although some research has shown that the average weight loss of some in OA is approximately 1 stone 8 pounds (9.9 kg or 21.8 lbs; Westphal, 1996). The OA literature states:

> We come to recognise that it is not how much we weigh or even how much we eat or don't eat that brings us to OA. It is the ways we have desperately tried to control our food, eating and weight. Some of us have tried to control our weight with extreme diets and exercise regimes. Some of us have gained and lost the same 20 or 25 pounds for many years, and the struggle has left us demoralised, frustrated and feeling like failures. Some of us are so afraid to get fat that we starve ourselves for periods of time, or we get rid of excess food by throwing up or purging with laxatives.

What a stark picture the OA members paint of themselves. An organization that can help overeaters to get off their spiral of despair and puts a stop to such destructive behaviour, however, surely deserves to be given great credit and, if their claims of weight loss are true – and if it lasts – then they are making progress along the right lines for them. It may not be an approach that suits all, however.

Do it yourself

WeightWatchers and Slimming World cost money so they are not an option for people on low incomes, although OA is a non-profit organization and its meetings may be attended for a minimal donation. The UK has lagged behind other countries in offering free help for people to direct them towards a better physical life-style, but there are signs that the situation is improving.

A few years ago, my own part of the UK, Scotland, was known (falsely) internationally for its hard-drinking and physically inactive population, living in poor social circumstances. We are the butt of many jokes about our bad eating habits, the classic one being that we eat deep-fried Mars bars and wash them down with a famously cheap 'tonic wine'. We Scots knew differently, of course, but it was hard to shake off the label when we promoted as our average citizen Rab C. Nesbitt with his string vest, headband and aversion to any physical exertion.

We are not as unfit and obese as we are popularly portrayed. Scotland has led the way in providing opportunities for her people to enjoy exercise freely and sociably. We have had the West Highland (112 miles, approximately 180 km) and Southern Upland Ways (235 miles, approximately 378 km), long walks across arguably the most beautiful countryside in Britain, for many years. They have been joined by the Scottish National Trail, from the Borders to Cape Wrath (a south to north walk of 470 miles, approximately 756 km) in 2012, but there are dozens of others. Simply look up walks in Scotland on the Internet and marvel how many there are. Of course, England, Wales and Northern Ireland provide similar services. Throughout the British Isles today, local and national authorities have provided marvellous walks that are open to everyone who fancies a day, week or even month or more of really pleasurable activity alongside others who are of like mind. Lifelong friendships have started on these routes.

Glasgow – yes the same city in which the fictional Rab C. Nesbitt lives – has established cycleways separated from the roads so that its citizens can cycle to work from the suburbs. My son Alasdair, now in his forties, cycles every day the seven miles from his home to Central Railway Station through parks and alongside the Clyde just to get to work. He isn't alone. Indeed, he is among hundreds of enthusiastic commuting cyclists.

To the south of Glasgow there is another network of walking and cycle tracks that snake into the largest area of wind turbines in Europe, a moorland more than 9 miles (15 km) across. On Boxing Day morning 2012, I and my son-in-law, another Alastair (slightly different spelling), walked his dog for 4 miles (8 km) over the moor, under and past the turbines, past small lochs and streams, meeting dozens of other post-Christmas exercisers on the way. We were just walking for the joy of it, in the crisp, dry air, enjoying the company of Linnhe the dog and the pleasure of meeting and greeting our fellow walkers and cyclists. This isn't an image of Glasgow that the rest of Britain recognizes.

My point is that if underprivileged and socially deprived Glasgow can do it, so can every other city. I'm sure that wherever you live in Britain, your city or town has organized walking and cycling tracks that you can use, not far from your home. Even if you are a sloth and don't feel like stirring yourself, you *can* follow my example.

Here I must make my own my personal confession. I am naturally a sloth. My parents were sloths, too. For as long as I can remember, they were overweight and they eventually paid for it by succumbing to the complications of their obesity. By the time I was 30, I was well on my way to following them. Working full time in medical practice had left me little time for leisure and, in the few hours I had when I was off duty, I tended to sleep. I gradually put on weight, so that I gained 2 stone (12.7 kg) in my first two years as a doctor.

A routine blood test (for life insurance – I was not ill) shocked me. I was clearly on my way to developing type 2 diabetes. It was a life-changing day as I then forced myself to become more physically active and eat less. In fact, the first thing led easily to the second. The more I moved about, the less I ate. Within a few months, my blood tests were back to normal and I had lost the extra weight.

It wasn't easy to change to begin with. There were many days when I couldn't be bothered to go outside, but I forced myself to do it. I had the advantage of having countryside on my doorstep and two young children to take with me. After the first month or so, my feelings changed. I felt that I couldn't pass a day without at least half an hour of walking and enjoying the outdoors. I looked forward to these times and the company of not just my children but also other friends who were walking enthusiasts. Exercise was no longer a chore, but a pleasure. I was no longer a sloth but a fidget and I haven't looked back.

So, sloths and fidgets are not immutably sloths or fidgets. If you see exerting yourself as a chore or a bother, you can change. You may have to be patient – the change will not happen over-night – but please persist. If you can get over that first hump – the feeling you can't be bothered – tell yourself, 'You can do it' and get like-minded friends or family to support you. It is a lot easier, and much more sociable and pleasurable, to increase your exercise levels if you do it with a trusted and likeable friend or friends.

Sport

One way to get into exercise with friends is to take up a sport. If you groan at this possibility, then it is probably not for you, but do read on.

All sorts of physical activity will make you fitter and if you find that doing things on your own is boring, then do consider taking up a sport. Taking part in sport not only means that you get involved in events but also you train for them, on a regular and structured basis. It is a good discipline for keeping you going when you feel like flagging. This is especially the case if you are the type of person who doesn't want to let the other members of your team or group down, so you force yourself to train even at times when the sloth in you raises its ugly head.

You will not be alone. More than 40 per cent of men and more than 31 per cent of women, aged 16 to 35 years, in England and

Wales were recorded as taking part in at least one sport at least
once a week between 1997 and 2006. The Brits are well behind the
Australians, 48 per cent of whom take part in sport three or more
times a week.

Being sporty is certainly good for your future as, in making
you fit, it significantly lessens your risk of early death. Dr L. B.
Andersen and colleagues (2000) followed two groups of adults for
14 years. Half were moderately active and half were active sportsmen and women. The sporty group were significantly less likely to
die in middle age than the non-sporty and lived longer and more
healthily into older age.

Which sport you choose doesn't matter, but the best evidence so
far (only because more people take part in it than in other sports) is
for five-a-side football. The Scandinavian group led by Dr P. Krustrup (2010) reported on adults (men and women) playing three-,
four- or five-a-side football two or three times a week for three to
four months. None had previously played the game and all were
new to strenuous exercise. All their medical indications of good
health, such as blood pressure, pulse rates, blood lipid levels and
tests for future diabetes, osteoporosis and lung function, improved
considerably.

Fears that starting to take up sport might injure you shouldn't
put you off. The disadvantages of injuries are very much less than
the benefits of the increase in fitness. Results like the above con-
tributed to the decision, in 2012, of the National Institute for
Health and Care Excellence (NICE) in England, Wales and Northern Ireland to advise, in a letter it sent out to general practitioners,
for them to 'prescribe' physical and sports activities for their unfit
patients. The Scots set up their ActiveScotland website for doctors
and their patients to find opportunities for sport and exercise
nearby. Doctors are being trained in how to advise their patients
as to what is the best type of exercise to suit them. Nurses and
physiotherapists are involved, too, as are a new breed of specialized medics, the 'exercise physiologists'.

It is early days yet, but the enthusiasm with which these new
initiatives have been greeted and their positive early results have
been heartening. Some of the initiatives, however, have led to surprising, even shocking, conflict between the experts about how

much we need to drink when taking exercise seriously. Do we need to avoid dehydration at all costs or is overhydration more of a problem? You may be surprised and even shocked by what the next chapter reveals about this subject.

4

Hydration intelligence

Imagine you have been enrolled as a helper at a marathon. You are standing at the 20-mile (32-km) post and a runner is staggering towards you, not able to stand up straight, obviously in distress. You move towards him, offering support, but he brushes you off. In fact, he is quite aggressive towards you and your colleagues until he falls to the ground. He then admits that he has a severe headache. He says he has been drinking plenty of water throughout the race and reaches for his sports drink bottle for some more. Do you let him drink or do you take the bottle from him?

It is crucial that you make the correct decision as the wrong one could have serious consequences or even be fatal.

For 30 years we have been bombarded with messages that we must avoid dehydration at all costs and drink plenty of water. Who hasn't heard that we should drink 3½ pints (2 litres) of water a day, over and above that in our food, to keep healthy? That we shouldn't wait until we are thirsty before we have a drink?

Is there a scientific basis for these claims? If there is, it is difficult to find. The 'drink a lot of fluids a day' movement started in the 1960s with Dr Robert Cade, a kidney specialist from the University of Florida. Dr Cade was worried sportsmen and -women might become dehydrated during their overexertions and he developed a 'sports drink' that would not only prevent dehydration but also supply the salts, minerals and sugars that they used up. It was called Gatorade™, after the local American Football team, the Gators.

From those small beginnings came a huge industry devoted to keeping sportsmen and women well hydrated and supplied with all the nutrients they needed. Other such sports drinks followed and, now, every exercising and sporting event is accompanied by a ubiquitous bottle of water or sports drink. Schoolchildren playing football are offered drinks every 20 minutes or so by their coaches, with extra water at half-time. Gone are the days of having half an orange and then getting straight back to it.

So, the answer is obvious, isn't it? Our man at the 20-mile (32-km) post needs a bit more water to revive him. He just hasn't been replenishing his fluids fast enough to keep up with what he has lost.

Wrong. You could kill him if you added yet more water to his system. He is showing all the signs – the aggression, confusion, weakness, poor coordination and headache – of overhydration. It is important to recognize these signs because, if you didn't, you would be a danger to the runner. His brain is swelling, so extra water may push the base of his brain down into the hole in the base of the skull that leads to the spinal cord. This is called 'coning', which is fatal if not immediately relieved.

This isn't a trivial matter, nor is it rare. Overhydration has been linked to at least 16 deaths and 1600 marathon runners becoming critically ill and needing intensive care (Cohen, 2012). Dehydration is much less serious, being easily reversed by drinking when you become thirsty, then stopping once you feel you have had enough. Drinking large amounts of extra fluids when you do not need to, however, is not helpful, does not improve your fitness or health and, as we have seen, can threaten your life.

Professor Arthur Siegel, of Harvard University and adviser to the Boston marathon, says there is no evidence that anyone doing a marathon has ever died from dehydration. 'Fluid is freely available in the races should the runner need to drink – they are not stranded in a desert with no access to fluids', he says (Cohen, 2012).

Professor Timothy Noakes (2012), of Cape Town University and the Sports Science Institute of South Africa, agrees with him. He states that dehydration, 'is a normal biological response to exercise. You lose water, you get thirsty, you drink. End of story.'

Whether or not we get thirsty during exercise, Professor Noakes explains, depends on how much we have sweated. Sweat is mostly water with a little salt (less salt than is proportionally in our blood and tissues), so sweating leads to a rise in sodium in the blood, which our brain senses and reacts to by making us thirsty in order to restore the balance. The thirstier we are, the less effectively we can exercise, which makes us exercise less, thereby conserving water. As soon as we drink enough to lose the thirst, the balance is back to normal and we can exercise more efficiently again.

This means that we always drink just enough, not too much.

We don't have a physical mechanism for coping with water overload, so there is no biological drive to make us 'overdrink'. Drinking more than we need to can disturb the delicate relationship between our body's fluid volume and our kidneys so that, paradoxically, athletes who have drunk too much water can still be thirsty and take in even more, leading to a vicious circle that underlies the deaths and emergencies that have affected so many people running marathons.

Professor Noakes stresses that there is barely any risk that dehydration will occur in athletes in an endurance event when there is plenty of water to drink on the way. Only when our total body water is reduced by 15 per cent, as happens when we are lost in a desert without water for more than a couple of days, do we lose control of our muscles. In contrast, overhydration by as little as 2 per cent will produce serious symptoms that need to be reversed urgently. For example, our runner from the beginning of this chapter would be given a strong intravenous salt solution drip to reduce his confusion, headache and muscle tone and encourage the kidneys to excrete as urine the extra volume of water to reduce his water overload.

The deaths and serious emergencies due to overhydration occur regardless of whether the drinks are simply water or 'sports' drinks. They are entirely due to the extra volume of water in the body.

In the past, the manufacturers of sports drinks have tried to claim that the problem of overhydration arises from drinking plain water and sports drinks are designed to avoid such dangerous falls in sodium levels. Professor Christopher Almond (2005), of Boston Children's Hospital, the lead author of the biggest study yet of marathon runners, financed not by industry but by the American National Institutes of Health, came to a different conclusion. He found that no such protection was given by sports drinks: he was very definite that it was the volume of the fluids alone that the runners had drunk, not their composition, that caused the problem:

The available evidence indicates that the most effective way to prevent hyponatremia (low blood sodium levels) during marathon running is to avoid a positive fluid balance.

In other words, drink just enough, as you need it, not before, to relieve your thirst and keep you from feeling thirsty.

I don't wish here to enter the massive row that has developed between industry and medical academics about the value and dangers of sports drinks and overuse of fluids in athletes, as this isn't a book on athletics. If you wish to read an independent review of them, please look up Deborah Cohen's (2012) article in the *British Medical Journal* and read the commentary there by Professor Noakes. You will be shocked by the way big business, promoting sports drinks and bottled water, it would seem, has manipulated the evidence (most of it poor) on the complexities of the ways in which our bodies deal with the fluids we drink.

What has all this stuff about fluid balance in endurance athletes to do with obesity and losing weight? Actually, quite a lot. The huge advertising and promotional campaigns behind sports drinks for athletes have spilled over into the slimming world. Sports drinks are commonly viewed as 'healthy' and, as such, harmless. If you are exercising regularly with the aim of losing weight, you will naturally want to replenish the fluids that you have lost and what better way than to do so by having a sports drink? If it is healthy, the rationale goes, it can't pile on the fat.

Sadly, that isn't correct. Approximately 18-fl oz (500-ml) bottles of the three most popular sports drinks contain much more sugar than you might think – from just over ½ oz to just over 1 oz (17.5 to 30 g). To put that into context, would you consider putting from 4½ to 7½ teaspoons of sugar in your cup of tea? Yet, more than a quarter of American parents (and probably the same proportion in the UK) believe that sports drinks are healthy for children.

The Robert Wood Johnson Foundation (2012) in the USA was so worried by the probable link between sports drinks and rising obesity levels in America, its main report stated that:

the increased consumption of sports drinks in recent years is of growing concern for parents, health professionals and public health advocates.

New York City's mayor, Michael Bloomberg, proposed in 2012 a ban on supersized bottles of soft drinks, including sports drinks, because of strong evidence that they are a prime cause of obesity in children and adults. As one commentator wrote, people are being convinced that if you drink a sports drink it will look after your body without you having to break out into a sweat.

In the UK, there is a battle raging, too. When the government tried to levy value-added tax on sports drinks, the UK Specialist Nutrition Alliance – supported by the drinks industry – countered with (quoted in Noakes' commentary alongside Cohen's article, 2012):

> You complain about obesity then charge us to live a healthy lifestyle – why penalise individuals for choosing to use products designed to maintain health and vitality which ultimately help reduce the burden on the already stretched and under resourced NHS? We are sitting on a diabetes and obesity time bomb.

So, do sports drinks reduce the risk of diabetes and obesity or actually increase it? Professor Noakes is in no doubt. He tells athletes that if they avoid sports drinks, they will get thinner and run faster.

The same message applies to you if you are simply trying to lose excess weight. There is no need for you to buy expensive drinks or drink to a strict programme, regardless of whether or not you are thirsty. Just drink when you need to, enough to stop your thirst, then drink again when you become thirsty again. Water is enough for you – you will get all your other nutrients from your food, which is what the next chapter is about. Before that, however, I must mention alcohol.

Alcohol

In 1991, Dr Serge Renaud, the Director of the French National Institute for Health and Medical Research in Lyon, was invited to appear on the US television programme *60 Minutes*. Its host, Morley Safer, asked him why the French had fewer heart attacks than did people living in similarly developed countries, such as the USA. He replied, 'I think it is the alcohol'. He ended the interview by raising a glass of red wine to his lips and saying, 'The protection of the French from heart disease may rest in this inviting glass.'

That statement, watched and heard by millions, was the start of the world's acceptance that alcohol is not simply a drug that can be abused but also a substance that can actually protect people from heart disease. Within a few weeks of the *60 Minutes* broadcast, sales of red wine in the USA rose by 40 per cent. The UK's wine sales followed the same upward curve and have continued to rise ever since.

The message has become universal: red wine, drunk in the French style, along with meals, should replace beers and spirits as the main way of consuming alcohol.

All sorts of reasons have been given for its benefits. Dr Renaud believed that polyphenols, found in the skin and pips of red grapes, were the secret heart-preserving ingredients that made red wine different from other forms of alcohol. Polyphenols, he and his colleagues discovered, alter cholesterol levels beneficially.

Research into red wine's properties by others has blossomed and the buzzword became resveratrol, found not only in red wine but also in green tea and apples, among other fruits and vegetables. Laboratory animals given resveratrol lived longer and with less heart disease than their peers. It seemed a simple matter to purify it and give it to humans, too.

Doubts arose when it was found that to get enough resveratrol from wine to protect our hearts would take many bottles a day – so many that we would quickly die from alcohol poisoning long before we could prove that we had been protected from having a heart attack. Sadly, the numbers of deaths from alcohol-related diseases have skyrocketed since the red wine revolution of the 1990s, far outweighing any obvious benefit of it in reducing incidences of heart attack or stroke.

Was Dr Renaud so wrong? No. He had hoped to promote the *sensible* use of alcohol, but what actually happened was that his message inadvertently opened the floodgates to alcohol misuse. Alcohol-related deaths have climbed from around seventh in our national statistics in the 1960s to third now (after high blood pressure and smoking).

While Dr Renaud's work involved persuading people to drink more red wine, it produced a strong backlash among doctors who had to deal with alcohol-related diseases. Even the French government didn't like his message, despite the increase in revenue it brought to France, as he had used government funding to promote alcohol. Government spokesmen declared that, 'in our country, as far as health is concerned, wine is alcohol and alcohol is abuse'.

The British became involved in the discussion as a result of doctors working with Professor Roger Williams of King's College Hospital London, whose studies in the 1970s of the drinking habits of people entering the hospital's liver unit (as he told me in a personal communication when I was working with him in 1975) mapped out precisely how much alcohol we could consume before we began to be at higher than average risk of liver and brain disease. The original advice hasn't changed much in the last 30 years, but our drinking habits have.

Forgive me for using Scotland as an example again, but we have the most closely scrutinized statistics on alcohol, confirming our popular stereotype. In 1960, Scotland had one of the lowest rates of death from cirrhosis of the liver in Western Europe; now it has one of the highest.

I believe that two changes in our society have led to this massive increase in misery:

- alcoholic drinks cost much less, proportionally, than they did 50 years ago
- the rules on the sale of alcohol and where and when it can be drunk have been relaxed, making it far easier now to drink up to and beyond the recommended number of units than it was.

The UK as a whole reflects the experience of the Scots. The advice is for women to drink fewer than 14 units of alcohol a week and for men to drink fewer than 21. This isn't to say that you should drink up to these limits, but, if you drink more, you are putting yourself at significantly greater risk than average of dying from liver or brain disease due to alcohol. These limits amount to a massive 48 pints (27.3 litres) of 40 per cent vodka in a year. That is roughly 3½ pints (2 litres) of vodka or 5 bottles of wine a month.

Sounds a huge amount to me, but you may think differently, because the average adult Briton drinks the equivalent of nearly 59 pints (33.4 litres) a year. Consider that this is the total sales of booze divided by the whole adult population, many of whom don't drink at all, so those who do drink are consuming more than that. The average drinker, then, must be getting through a great deal more than the equivalent of 70 pints (40 litres) of vodka.

One unit of alcohol is a little less than 3 tsp (10 ml) of pure ethanol. Beers contain from 4 to 8 per cent alcohol, wines around 12 to 13 per cent (they used to contain 8 to 10 per cent), fortified wines more than 15 per cent and spirits around 40 per cent. I'll do the calculations for you. In today's terms, 14 units (the upper limit for women) is easily reached by a single glass of wine a day or a large measure of spirits on 4 or 5 days a week. Add half again to calculate the figures for men. Drinkers today rarely limit themselves to such apparently small amounts and are often shocked by their totals when they use a diary to note them down.

The other misapprehension among regular drinkers is that liver and brain disease only happen to alcoholics – people who regularly drink to get drunk – but that's not so. The whole point about the research carried out by King's College Hospital is that they can arise in people who have never been the worse for drink – all it needs is for your drinking to be a little more than your weekly limit.

Of course, alcohol is not the only ingredient of wines, beers and spirits. There is plenty of sugar in them, too, particularly if you add a mixer to your spirits – ginger ale to a whisky or brandy or tonic to your gin or cola to your vodka adds quite a few usually uncounted calories to your total intake.

So what advice are we left with for people who need to lose weight?

- Always keep close control of your alcohol intake.
- Don't drink that second glass.
- Try to do without for three days a week.

- Never binge: the evidence is accumulating that binge drinking at the weekends is at least as dangerous to your long-term health prospects as regular drinking every day. Preferably restrict your alcohol to mealtimes, so that you enjoy it slowly as you take time over your food.
- Make it a special event, not a routine that you must have a certain drink at a specific time every day.

That way, you will enjoy it more in the long run and that long run may be longer and more enjoyable as a result.

5

Nutritional intelligence

Eating

'Diet' is a four-letter word. As a rule I don't use it when advising people on weight problems. In the sense that the word means restricting types, combinations, quantities and timing of food in order to solve a medical problem such as obesity, it is a mistaken, sometimes even dangerous, course to follow. Eating should be a pleasure, not medication, and diets imposed on us to persuade us to lose weight are surely a form of medicine, in that they are treatment for a medical condition. That isn't a healthy attitude.

We eat, obviously, to survive. We need to swallow food and drink to supply our body with all that is needed to keep us healthy and active. We are social human beings as well, however, and eating is far more than simply a mechanism for fuelling our activities until we become hungry again.

Bear with me as I refer once more to our prehistory as hunter-gatherers. Our ancestors were omnivores – that is, we ate what we could find, animal or vegetable, and our digestive systems developed in line with those habits. We have teeth that are designed to cut and grind meats and seeds; we have a gut designed to deal with animal and vegetable material; and we have a series of digestive enzymes that have developed to cope with all sorts of food. (We do lack cellulase – the enzyme that grazing animals have to break down grasses and other raw green vegetables – but that is a minor point.)

So, in one way, we should be prepared to eat everything that we can digest, because that is how we have evolved. As hunter-gatherers, we had the means to digest animal and plant material and functioned better if we could find both. In fact, our survival as a species probably depended on our ancestors being able to do exactly that.

Modern humans, however, are much more than hunter-gatherers: we are social animals and, for many generations, in every society, we have made a habit of sharing our food and eating together. Most societies make eating the highlight of their day and this is seen especially in Italy, Spain and Greece, the northern Mediterranean countries. When following their traditional diet, as explained in Chapter 2, Italians, Greeks and Spaniards enjoy their food so much they rarely 'diet', yet remain, on the whole, slim and fit.

So, the theme that we can see running through this chapter is to eat wisely and happily and make it a part of your life that you can enjoy. Going on any diet that is a chore is never an answer. Nor are systems of eating that measure, weigh and exclude foods as, when you adopt such an artificial approach to eating, enjoyment becomes secondary and your good intentions begin to melt away.

You will gather from this that I am not going to endorse any of the faddy diets that seem to be the main reason for the existence of many women's (and a few men's) magazines. There are no miracle diets.

I will write about individual diets later in this chapter, but, first, let me explain about digestion and how the body deals with food. Once they are understood it will become clearer why faddy and other 'diets' can be at least nonsense or worse, actively harmful.

Proteins, fats and carbohydrates

Our three main foodstuffs are made up of proteins, fats and carbohydrates (sugars and starches). When we swallow food, we trigger the release of enzymes that break down (digest) the complex chemistry of each type of food into its basic elementary parts, or, molecules. The digestion process begins in the mouth, where saliva starts to work on starches and complex sugars, continues in the stomach, where proteins start to be broken down into peptides, and then in the small intestine, where enzymes from the pancreas and bile complete the process, producing the endpoints of digestion – glucose from the carbohydrates, amino acids from the proteins and fatty acids from the fats.

Only then can these substances pass through the gut wall, to be taken up by the circulation to the liver, which then starts the process of building them up again into the proteins, carbohydrates and fats that we need, ready to be dispersed to our tissues and organs. They are all *our* proteins, fats and carbohydrates, bearing very little direct relationship to the ones we have eaten.

We make our own kind of protein from the building blocks of the proteins we ate in the form of meat or fish. Likewise, our livers build up the types of fats our organs need from the fats and carbohydrates we ate or drank. We have human fat – not pig fat or vegetable oils – in our fat storage tissues. All the starches we eat – from potatoes, flour and rice, for example – are converted into glucose, which is the only carbohydrate we can use directly for energy. The only other carbohydrate we use is glycogen, which our muscles use as a store of energy. It is a slightly more complex molecule than glucose that almost instantaneously converts into glucose when the muscles need it. Once we have used up our glucose and glycogen, we then have to turn to our fat stores to find a source of our energy.

All these processes are constantly going on inside us, independently of each other. Knowing this, it makes little sense, as some diet moguls proclaim, to separate some forms of food – even less, just one from the others to create a specialized 'diet'. There is no biological or biochemical basis for doing so, despite the claims of commercially minded 'experts'.

There is one overriding fact to remember about eating: if we eat more than we need for the energy we are using, we will store the extra as fat. To do so we need a vast number of fat storage cells, which are mostly present in a thick layer under our skin. Some of us are 'pears' – storing the fat around our hips and bottoms – while others are 'apples' – storing it around our middles. Years of overeating and/or underexercising eventually make us tubby or wobbly. It doesn't take much for this to happen. Just one extra snack a day can cause you to put on 11 lbs (5 kg) or so of fat in a year round your waist, bottom and hips. Do it for 20 years and you will be 220 lbs (100 kg) heavier.

I'd bet that, as you are reading this, you aren't near to 220 lbs (100 kg) over your optimum weight. It's more likely you are around 44 lbs (20 kg) heavier than you should be. That's only a fifth of a snack a day too much – a very small extra, taken over many years. So, you can see, determining to eat a little bit less every day will definitely help. From the previous chapter, you will have learned that it is easy to lose excess weight by increasing your exercise levels. So, combine both the slight change in your regular eating habits with a little more exertion every day and you will have started in motion your winning formula.

Here, though, is where it becomes complicated again. You would have had to have lived on Mars for the last 30 years to have missed the message that being fat gives you a higher than normal risk of dying early from a heart attack or stroke. It seems simple: the fatter you are, in the sense that you have a bigger waistline or hip measurement, the more likely it is that you will keel over early from heart failure, a heart attack or stroke. The odd thing is that this so-called simple fact is very difficult to prove, if you can prove it at all. There are plenty of fat people who live long and apparently healthy lives. My favourite examples are Winston Churchill and Patrick Moore of *The Sky at Night* fame, who were obviously grossly obese yet lived happily into their late eighties. Conversely, there are plenty of thin people who suffer one or more heart attacks and/or a stroke before they reach old age.

Why should there be so many exceptions to the rule? Is it what we eat rather than how much? Are some people simply programmed genetically to be fat and, separately, to die young, while others are destined to reach old age regardless of their shape? We are only beginning to find the answers to these questions.

Let us return to ghrelin and leptin, which were mentioned in Chapter 1. We will start with ghrelin.

If your stomach has been empty for a few hours, it decides to make you fill it again by secreting ghrelin into your bloodstream. The brain uses this signal to make you feel hungry, so that you organize getting something to eat. As soon as you start to swallow food, the ghrelin levels fall and your hunger begins to diminish. That feeling is reinforced by the arrival of leptin in your blood.

Leptin is a curious hormone. It isn't produced in your stomach, but by your fat cells – the very ones that you have accumulated around your tummy and/or hips and bottom. It rises in response to the rising levels of fats and glucose in your body that are the consequence of your having eaten. When the brain registers these rising leptin levels in your blood, it shuts down your appetite. At the same time, the extra leptin removes excess fat from the bloodstream, causing the body to burn some of it off and divert the rest to the fat cells.

To summarize, ghrelin makes you hungry, making you eat and start to process all the nutrients in your food, and leptin makes you feel full, lose your appetite and store any excess of fat in those specialized fat cells.

Yet, things are not that simple for some of us. For most, the ghrelin–leptin cycle seems a perfect way to deal with hunger and satiation, but it seems to be different if you are overweight or obese. Common sense, for example, might lead you to think that obesity could be caused by either a higher and longer ghrelin response (making you feel hungrier for longer) or a lower or delayed leptin response (so you don't lose your appetite as fast as usual or at all when you eat).

On the contrary, obese people have much higher than average leptin levels over longer than average periods. It seems that their bodies have tried hard in the past to stop them eating too much or for too long and have stepped up the leptin production to achieve this. Sadly, the constantly high leptin level makes the brain lose its sensitivity to the hormone, so the feeling of satiation that you would expect does not happen.

There is a problem with ghrelin, too. Overweight and obese people who start to lose weight by eating less – I reluctantly have to use the word diet here – start to make more ghrelin, so that they become *hungrier* than before. It seems that the body doesn't like the lower food intake and responds by trying to make you step it up, to replace the fat you have lost. You would think, too, that obese people, with their reputedly greater than average appetite, would have higher levels of ghrelin, but they don't. In fact, their ghrelin levels are *lower* than normal, so it is assumed that the brain in overweight people is much more sensitive to the hormone than is the brain in someone of standard weight. Thus, in the overweight, smaller amounts of ghrelin induce a more potent hunger response than is usually the case.

The story for ghrelin is even more complicated. There are reports, not yet confirmed for sure by further studies, but which seem convincing, that people who have had bariatric surgery (removal of much of the stomach to reduce obesity) produce much less ghrelin than they did before the operation. That seems to explain part of the success of such surgery as patients who have had it report having a much smaller appetite than before. It is true that the mechanical shrinking of the stomach makes them feel fuller despite having less food, but they see that as a separate feeling from that of their loss of appetite. It is just as well, because if they had kept their original appetite, they would be in danger of eating too much for their new smaller stomach, with probably dire consequences for them.

To summarize, we eat because we produce ghrelin in our stomachs and that makes us hungry. We stop eating because we lose the feeling of hunger as a consequence of falling levels or ghrelin and rising levels of leptin, produced by our fat cells. Our livers transform the foodstuffs we have eaten into human fats and proteins. The leptin helps to push the fats into the tissues that need them and the excess into our fat cells for storage.

Now to the next piece in the puzzle. In the meantime, another hormone, insulin, has been processing the glucose we have accumulated from the sugars and starches we have eaten. It is produced by the pancreas in response to the rise in blood glucose levels that occur following a meal containing sugars and starches. The main purpose of insulin is to distribute the glucose to all our tissues and organs as every cell in the body uses glucose for its energy needs. Normally insulin is exceptionally efficient at its job, starting to lower blood glucose levels within minutes. Any excess glucose that is not needed for immediate energy purposes is converted in the liver into fat and passed on to those fat storage cells that are already, thanks to leptin, mopping up the excess fat from the food we have eaten.

Clearly, leptin, ghrelin and insulin work in close cooperation with each other, regulating what can be used for energy purposes and what can be stored. Although that system of cooperation works well when we are of normal weight, it begins to break down when we become obese. Perhaps this part of the book is the most important for you to understand, because it is the rational basis on which, if you are overweight, you can start your new way of living.

I posed a couple of questions a few pages ago.

- Why do some people keep well despite being obese?
- Is it the quantity or the type of food we eat that matters?

The key to answering them lies in those fat storage cells and how the way we eat and what we eat affects them.

It is revolutionary, but one explanation for being an apple or a pear is that becoming either shape actually protects you from heart attack and stroke – or at least postpones them. It has been hard for a doctor like me, who has been trying to help overweight and obese patients all my life, to accept that sometimes being fat can be better for them than many of the treatments (mainly diets and some forms of surgery) designed to help them to lose weight. The accepted truism is anything that will help fat people shed their extra weight must be good. That is patently wrong, but it will take a little more of me describing the technical stuff to explain it to you. Please bear with me as I do this in the next few paragraphs.

Let us get rid of the apple versus pear argument first. It has been accepted that 'apples' fare worse than 'pears' in terms of their risk of early death from heart attack or stroke. I wish I could find good evidence for that often repeated statement, but I can't. The risk of dying early if you are overweight and either shape depends much more on the amount of your extra weight than where under the skin it is distributed. The heavier you are, on the whole, the greater the risk, if, of course, you forget Sirs Winston and Patrick. Losing excess weight is good for you, regardless of where on your body you have lost it from. How you lose it, though, and how you gained it in the first place do matter.

Let us start with the fact that it is never the fat around your tummy or on your hips or rear that kills you. Obese people die instead from the fat that is deposited in the walls of their blood vessels – in the brain or heart or even around the abdominal internal organs. The new belief among experts in cardiology, neurology and vascular diseases is that, for many people, the deposits of fat around the midriff, hips and rear are *saving* their lives as they are better there than elsewhere. Indeed, some treatments designed to remove such areas of fat have the effect of shifting future fat deposits to the alternative store sites of the heart, gut and brain, but I'll come to that later.

Metabolic syndrome

A major factor that seems to differentiate people who die from their obesity from those who don't is the presence of 'metabolic syndrome'. Not all obese people have it, but those who do are at extreme risk of serious health complications, including early death. Very few thin people develop it, but those who do are at the same high risk of early death as their heavier peers.

Remember the Pima described in Chapter 1? The fact that most of them developed diabetes and many of them died young strongly suggests that they had metabolic syndrome and it was from complications of it that they died. The huge rise in the numbers of people with type 2 diabetes (remember the 15-fold rise worldwide in the last two generations) has coincided exactly with the rise in obesity. Also, it is far higher than the already steep three-fold rise in the world's population as a whole. The life expectancy of people with poorly controlled type 2 diabetics, whether they are fat or thin, is shorter than that of obese people who do not have diabetes. Perhaps Winston Churchill and Patrick Moore were just lucky – they were not genetically programmed to develop it. Perhaps they ate more wisely than most, even if they ate too much to keep slim. The sort of food you have eaten over the years to get to the weight you are now really does seem to matter.

In metabolic syndrome, there are three threatening problems: high blood pressure, type 2 diabetes and a high total cholesterol (and therefore blood fat) level. It makes those who have it much more prone than average – and other obese people without it – to have a heart attack and stroke. Enter Doctors Roger Unger and Philipp Scherer, specialists in diabetes at the Southwestern Medical Center in Dallas, which is part of the University of Texas. They are world leaders in the new knowledge we have of metabolic syndrome. They told the *New Scientist*'s Andy Coghlan (2010) that, 'obesity protects the body from the effects of overeating by providing somewhere safe to deposit the dietary deluge of fat and sugar, which in excess is toxic to many body tissues'.

How did they arrive at a conclusion that, in the light of the accepted direct relationship between obesity and early death from a heart attack and stroke, seems wholly irrational? They based it on the work they have done on those fat cells or, more to the point, the absence of fat cells, in animals and humans, and the relationship they have with the initiation of metabolic syndrome.

Drs Unger and Scherer bred a strain of mice with very low numbers of fat storage cells. When they gave them a high-fat diet, the mice did not become fat, but they did develop the mouse equivalent of human metabolic syndrome. Amazingly, there are people who have inherited a condition in which they have no fat storage cells. They are thin but healthy – unless they eat large amounts of fat. Then they, like the mice, develop metabolic syndrome.

The Southwestern Medical Center team reasoned that, in humans who have started to develop metabolic syndrome, all the fat cells are crammed full of so much fat that they cannot take up any more. The fat cells then begin to die off and the fats that were stored inside them then spill back into the blood circulating the body, from where they are taken up by the liver, pancreas and heart. The damage the fats do to these vital organs leads to the high blood pressure, diabetes and the high levels of cholesterol in the blood that denote metabolic syndrome.

Drs Unger and Scherer add that leptin plays a part in the genesis of metabolic syndrome, too. You will recall that leptin causes the body to burn off fat and to direct any excess into the fat cells. To begin with, therefore, it is a protective hormone. As we grow older, however, leptin becomes less effective. With age, if we are obese, our fat cells begin to 'leak' fats back into the blood, as mentioned above, first helping to initiate metabolic syndrome and then worsen it.

Dr Preeti Kishore (Coghlan, 2010) and her team at the Albert Einstein College of Medicine in New York have proposed a mechanism to explain how the extra fats in the bloodstream lead to metabolic syndrome. She found 30 volunteers who would allow her to inject fat equivalent to that found in a beefburger straight into their veins. Their bodies responded by producing a surge of a substance entitled plasminogen activator inhibitor-1 (PAI-1).

PAI-1 has complex actions, all of which can be directly linked to metabolic syndrome. It makes cells less responsive to insulin, thereby helping to initiate diabetes, it promotes blood clotting, raising the risk of heart and brain disease, and is probably also linked to rising blood pressure.

The picture is becoming clear. As we put on weight, the cells that store fat start to fill up, leading to our broadening shape and increasing weight. They have huge, but not infinite, capacity, so many years may elapse before the trouble starts. Eventually, sooner in some people and later in others, the load of stored fat becomes too much and the cells begin to spill it back into the bloodstream. That process brings about the changes that lead to metabolic syndrome – the high blood pressure, high levels of cholesterol and diabetes that are the real and direct cause of the early deaths that occur in many obese people.

Given these facts, it becomes clear that the top priority for anyone with weight problems is not simply to reduce the waistline or become thinner. Rather, it is incumbent on us to try to do it without making the health risks worse.

Of course, a prime way to do this is to stop filling up the fat storage cells with more fat by eating sensibly and burning it up by exercising. Eating less, if you do eat too much, will also help to lower the flow of fats from the liver to the fat storage cells, but doing that alone without also exercising is unlikely to bring long-term success.

By now it has probably occurred to you that some approaches to losing weight are plainly wrong, counterproductive and even dangerous. The worst of them is liposuction. That involves sticking a rigid tube under the skin into the fat layer and applying suction, a bit like a vacuum cleaner, to remove it. It doesn't just remove the fat: it also removes the fat storage cells and, once they are gone, the body will not replace them. So, if, as some people do, they continue, after liposuction, to overload their meals with fat or sugars (remember, any excess of sugar is turned into fat), the body can no longer store it around the waist or in the buttocks or thighs. The fat will then go into and around the internal organs. It isn't difficult to work out that this is bad medicine and surgery.

Low-carbohydrate, high-protein diets, such as that originally promoted so successfully by Robert Atkins and copied in slightly different ways by many others, are as questionable as liposuction. I'll deal with them and other similar diets in the next few paragraphs, but first I'd like to concentrate on healthy eating.

It is worth repeating that if we expend exactly the same amount of energy as the amount of potential energy gained from digesting food we have taken in, we will stay at the same weight. If we eat less and burn off more in exercise, we will lose weight. If we eat more and exercise less, we will put it on. These are laws of physics, as well as of physicians.

So, to start with, we need to eat just enough to cover all our energy needs. We don't need to measure anything to know if we are doing it right – we simply have to weigh ourselves or put a tape measure around our waists and hips. In fact, a glance in the mirror is usually enough.

Let's start by declaring that we should eat when we feel hungry, take it slowly, enjoy what we eat and stop when we have had enough. Trust your ghrelin and leptin responses. Eating should be a pleasure that we look forward to. Think Italian – or Spanish or Greek. Vary what you eat widely. We are the first generation to enjoy vegetables and fruits fresh from all over the world all year round, so take advantage of the glorious spectrum of tastes that they offer. Above all, don't restrict the amount you eat so that you are always hungry, even if you believe it to be the fastest way to lose weight. If you do that you will reprogramme your leptin and ghrelin balance to give you a sharper appetite and keep the feeling going until you eventually eat something. You will delay the start of the feeling of satiation, ending your misery by eating more than before.

That's not all a starvation (let's call a spade a spade) diet will do for you. You become a hunter-gatherer again and force your body to think that it is in a time of famine. It has to adapt quickly in the only way it knows how: it sets up a mechanism that, for future times of glut, makes it much more efficient at storing fat. The fat cells become more sensitive to leptin, so they will be able to store more fat in the future as your actions have given it the message that this will be necessary.

At least as damaging is a process called adaptive thermogenesis, in which your body, in a response to the lower intake of food, resets the rate at which it expends energy during normal living to a slower level. M. Rosenbaum and R. L. Leibel (2010) wrote about this effect. They showed that if on a low-calorie diet you lose 10 per cent of your body weight, your body responds by shutting down your energy expenditure by a fifth to a quarter. That seems to be a permanent change, so if you gain weight again and want to resume dieting to lose it, you need to cut out far more calories than before to achieve the same weight loss. It is a vicious circle. Your future dieting, if it means lower than normal food intake, will be harder, make you feel hungrier, be even more damaging and far more difficult to keep up than before. With each bout of dieting, the circle turns once more.

That explains why 98 per cent of people who try low-calorie diets return to their former weight within 18 months and most of them carry on gaining. Our bodies don't like being constantly, or even intermittently, exposed to famine conditions and will go to extremes to overcome them. That isn't what you want and goes a long way to explaining why so many dieters fail.

A. J. Hill had the last word on such diets in 2004 in the *British Journal of Nutrition*. He wrote that, in 2002, 231 million Europeans had taken up diets in their efforts to lose weight. Only 1 per cent of them were successful. It is a strange result for a massive industry's efforts. Which other industry could remain viable if its main product experienced a 99 per cent failure rate?

'That's fine,' I can almost hear you say, 'but I don't want to starve. I'd like to try one of those diets that doesn't make me hungry, but concentrates on getting rid of my fat.'

There are plenty of them, of course. They all depend on avoiding a particular type of food and making up for the lack by increasing your intake of other foodstuffs. Robert Atkins was the most famous of these, with his low-carbohydrate, high-protein regimen. Atkins advocated eating as much as you liked of meat, cheese and eggs, but made you do without sugar, bread, pasta, fruit, vegetables and milk. The idea was that without sugars and starches, the body had to rely on burning fats for energy. That would, the theory went, deplete the fat stores with ease and without pain.

A little chemistry here. When we use glucose (from sugars and starches) for energy, it burns away to carbon dioxide and water, two substances that are easily disposed of in our breath and urine. Take glucose out of the equation and we have to burn fat instead. When we do, it breaks down into a ketone called acetone, which you may recognise as causing the sweet smell from the breath of someone with poorly controlled diabetes.

Ketones have become a buzzword in the dietary firmament, with minor starlets espousing ketone diets as the way to lose weight in magazine after magazine. They are still doing so years after the Atkins diet was finally shown to be a failure.

As I mentioned earlier, the results from the latest and largest study of low-carbohydrate, high-protein diets of 43,396 Swedish women over 15.7 years should put an end to such diets once and for all. The women were 'scored' for how rigidly they adhered to the diet and, for each tenth of an increase in their scores, the women had a rise of 5 per cent in their incidence of heart disease. Those who adhered most closely to the diet, with the highest scores, had a staggering 62 per cent increase in their incidence of heart attacks and stroke over the baseline of women not on the diet. A diet that kills you while you are losing weight is surely the final straw for artificial eating habits.

Why were the long-term results so bad for the women? Atkins had failed to take into account that his non vegetable and non fruit system led to reduced intakes of vitamins and minerals that meant they built up serious deficiencies over the months and years. Equally important, the excess of fats and proteins in his regimen led to exactly the same kinds of fatty deposits in their arteries that obese people have to minimize if they are to remain healthy. Atkins had prescribed the very opposite of what they needed.

So, the main message of this chapter is hardly sensational. It is that eating is good for you, if you do it in moderation and ensure you have great variety. We live in times where the opportunities to eat well and healthily have never been greater. Take advantage of them, but don't overdo it.

The 'don't overdo it' warning is needed more today than ever. We live in times when we are besieged every day by fantastic cookery programmes that extol the best in food and drink. Haute cuisine has become the norm – TV chefs share the same level of celebrity as footballers. Reality TV broadcasts competitions week after week involving young, amateur and professional chefs, all vying to become the 'Master' of their world. Millions try to emulate them in their homes and restaurants throughout the country have seriously upped their game in their efforts to compete with what their customers see on TV.

The result has been a staggering rise in the quality of the food we eat at home and when we go out to eat. Even ready meals have improved beyond belief. Although we are constantly told that we are in a time of austerity, far more of us are able to afford to eat out more often than we did a generation ago. The portions are larger and the food is richer and more varied. We are tempted by starters, main courses and desserts, washed down with glasses of wine, in good company and a welcoming, friendly and professional atmosphere. No wonder we overindulge, forgetting that we may have taken in enough in one evening to supply around four days worth of our normal energy needs.

If that applies to you and you need to lose weight, yet still want to enjoy yourself, why not settle for, say, two starters or a starter and a dessert or a single main course? How about just one glass of wine? Remember that one large glass of wine contains the equivalent in calories of two chocolate digestive biscuits, as well as nearly three units of alcohol, of course. A bottle of water on the table, so that you can alternate your slurps with a non-alcoholic (and non-calorific) sip or two, will keep you on the right lines, avoiding that feeling of guilt the next day.

Of course, you can shun all that high living and exist, according to some diet gurus, on cabbages. To cheer you up, I have in front of me as I write a full-page advertisement in a national newspaper extolling their virtues. 'At last,' it proclaims, 'the world famous cabbage soup diet is now available in a gel capsule.'

Cabbage soup, the advert informs us, 'is a natural weight loss aid used by men and women all round the world'. It admits, however, that not everyone is prepared to eat cabbage soup every day, so the company has 'developed a method of extracting all the goodness of cabbage soup and condensing it into a gel capsule without taste or aftertaste. The recommended dosage is 3 capsules a day.'

It goes on to say that cabbages have more vitamin C than oranges, great for strengthening the immune system and being one of the best antioxidants for reducing the free radicals in your body, which cause ageing. It adds that cabbage is very rich in glutamine – an amino acid that is useful for ensuring that our digestive system functions effectively.

It is difficult to substantiate these claims (and in any case the capsules are very expensive). For example, cooking cabbages to make the soup would certainly destroy its vitamin C. You would have to eat it raw to have a chance of absorbing the vitamin from the cabbage leaves, which raises the problem mentioned earlier of our not having the cellulase enzyme in our gut needed to break down the cell walls of the cabbage leaves to get at the vitamins inside. Rabbits have plenty of it, but we aren't rabbits. As for glutamine, we ingest masses of it from other sources. I can't find a report in the literature of any case of glutamine deficiency in humans and I don't know on what evidence the company bases its statement that it is useful for ensuring that our digestive system functions effectively. I assume that, after the company has processed the cabbage into a gel, it will still possess the magic ingredients, including those exciting antioxidants (to be discussed in Chapter 7), which it says will help people to lose weight, but I don't see anywhere in the advertisement a list of what the gel capsule actually contains. I certainly wouldn't endorse such diets to my patients.

6

Fasting intelligence

Despite what I said at the end of the previous chapter, it is a fact that people who are persuaded to try the kinds of odd ways to lose weight mentioned there do actually shed some weight in the first few weeks. It's clear, though, that the loss isn't due to any magic action the tablets or diet are having on the body; it is because, while on it, what is actually happening is you are fasting. You are eating too little other food to sustain your energy needs, so you lose weight. It is that old law of physics at work again.

You can't sustain a long fast, but fasting (the word sounds better than 'starving', which it actually is) could be beneficial in the long run, if you are careful to do it healthily. The 5:2 fasting diet, for example, fashionable in 2012–2013, has been criticized as a temporary fad, but may have a positive side, if practised responsibly, and make sense for some people, but certainly not all.

The idea, based on a principle known as intermittent fasting, is simple: eat what you feel like on five days a week, then fast – that is, eat minimally – on the other two. On your two fasting days, if you are a woman, you restrict yourself to a total count of no more than 500 calories in your food and drink choices. Men are allowed 600 calories. The two fasting days must not be consecutive – though some people do make them so – and, in the rest of the week, you can eat your fill of anything you fancy.

The idea, of course, is to replicate, as nearly as possible, the conditions we endured as hunter-gatherers. It uses the fact that we are still hunter-gatherers at heart. Our bodies have been attuned for millennia to odd days of hunger, so if we return to that pattern, albeit only for a day at a time, our bodies may readjust accordingly and make us slimmer and fitter.

Fasting isn't new, of course. Every religion endorses periods of fasting, mainly as an aid to greater clarity of thinking, but, behind so many religious traditions, like the holy month of Ramadan for Muslims, the Day of Atonement and Yom Kippur for Jews and Lent for Christians, have been health messages. Depriving yourself of food for a relatively short time was known to make you feel better, 'more alive', and help you think straight. Of course, ordinarily, unless you have an eating disorder, you can't keep up the fasting habit for a long period without feeling so hungry and stressed that you have to give it up.

There are people who manage to do it, such as, in the UK, the wonderful Fauja Singh, renowned for years for running the London Marathon. In 2012, he completed it at the age of 101 – all on what we would consider to be a starvation diet of no meat or fish, just small portions (too small, we ordinary mortals would think) of vegetables, lentils sprinkled with ginger, plus fruit, yogurt and brown bread.

There is evidence to show that fasting reduces levels of IGF-1 (an insulin-like growth factor, secreted in the liver in response to protein in the diet), which we use to speed up the rate at which cells burn up energy. Not only does fasting lower our own levels of IGF-1 but it also switches our body's activities from 'growth mode' to 'repair mode', in particular, 'switching on' the actions of genes that repair faulty DNA – the double helix code at the centre of all our cells. Low levels of IGF-1, in turn, may boost longevity.

Studies of mice by Professor Valter Longo and colleagues (Mosley, 2012), of Southern California's Longevity Institute, suggests that some mice (called Laron mice for reasons that will become clear in a moment), which lack the ability to respond to IGF-1, thus slowing down their metabolism, age more slowly than other mice. The same would appear to happen in humans.

Certain villagers in Ecuador, diagnosed with a rare genetic condition called Laron syndrome or Laron dwarfism, similarly cannot respond to IGF-1. They live longer than people in nearby villages, though, according to Professor Longo, not as long as they might, due to their proclivity for unhealthy habits, such as having a very fatty diet and smoking.

The problem, of course, is that we can't fast for long without becoming ill. If we starve ourselves for much longer than a day, our blood pressure will fall, blood glucose levels drop and metabolism slow down so that we don't feel like being active and definitely not 'full of life'. We become physically weaker and may even faint.

Dr Michael Mosley (2012) wrote about when he tried fasting in *The Telegraph*. After fasting for three days, he had lost more than 2 lbs pounds of fat, his resting blood glucose level had fallen steeply and, probably most importantly, his IGF-1 level (he had been struck by, and was obviously anxious about, how high it had been) had halved.

Dr Mosley found he coped better with the three-day fast than he had expected. He was hungry for a day, but his hunger eased off after that, even though he had only consumed black tea and coffee and water. Deciding that three days of fasting was too long, he then changed to the system of alternating the days of fasting promoted by Dr Krista Varady of Chicago's University of Illinois.

Dr Varady (Mosley, 2012) had volunteers fast on alternate days, restricting themselves to 600 calories on the fast days if they were men, 500 calories if they were women. That is interesting enough, but what is really fascinating is that she asked half of them to eat low-fat foods and the other half to eat high-fat foods, such as pizzas and lasagnes, on their non-fasting days. Her study therefore had two aims:

- to see how well the volunteers coped with fasting on alternate days;
- to see which group – on the high- or low-fat diet – would lose most weight.

All the volunteers coped well. Initially, those who had been allocated to the high-fat eating pattern were a little unhappy because they thought that they would lose less weight than the others. In fact, the two groups lost the same amount of weight and, more importantly, their blood tests showed that their risks of heart attack and stroke had diminished by the same amount throughout the study. Further, their LDL cholesterol levels had fallen, along with their blood pressure, regardless of what they had eaten on their non-fast days. Not surprisingly, Dr Varady and her very willing volunteers are continuing the trial, fasting on alternate days for at least another year, to study the long-term outcomes.

After meeting with Drs Longo and Varady, Dr Mosley decided to join the fun. Rather than follow the alternating days pattern, though, he decided on the slightly less demanding discipline of the 5:2 system. He chose Tuesdays and Thursdays as his fast days. At first, he wasn't sure how to divide up his 600 calories. Eating them all at once in the mornings made him too hungry later, but leaving having food until later made him too hungry in the mornings. So, he split them into two lots of 300 calories, eating at breakfast time and in the early evening. That seemed to work for him.

His fast day breakfast consists of two scrambled eggs, a slice of ham, water, green tea and black coffee. His evening meal comprises grilled fish and loads of vegetables. Not bad for a fast day!

On non-fast days, he reports, he and other 5:2 fasters as a whole don't take to overeating. So, after six weeks of adopting this 5:2 pattern, Dr Mosley had lost over a stone (6.3 kg) and was down to the weight he wanted to be – 12 stone (76 kg or 168 lbs). His blood glucose level, which had been bordering on the diabetic, had come down to well within the normal range. His blood cholesterol level had also fallen, from a level that was going to need him to take medication to one that was well below the 'risk' range. His IGF-1 level remained low throughout the time he followed the new way of eating – a significant pointer to his having a lower risk of heart disease and stroke.

He looks and feels better than before and has decided to stay on this 5:2 fast. For anyone who, like the good doctor, is overweight but otherwise healthy, it is difficult to see what harm can come from it, but it is still important to seek medical advice before embarking on it to ensure that is the case for you.

As with all such anecdotes, we should follow Dr Mosley's example with caution. It has obviously been good for him, but his is an individual example and, at the time of writing, there aren't that many studies of 5:2 fasting to give us a clear picture as to whether this would be the case for everyone, certain groups of people and so on.

A study at the University Hospital of South Manchester NHS Foundation Trust (Harvie et al., 2011) looked at 107 overweight women who either followed a balanced weight loss eating plan or a 5:2 fasting diet. The study found that the amount of weight lost was similar in both groups – just under a stone (6 kg or 13 lbs) – though those in the fasting group showed slightly better results in terms of their insulin and blood sugar levels. At the end of the study, however, only 58 per cent of those on the fasting diet planned to continue, whereas 85 per cent of those following a balanced diet said they would.

A study of 30 obese women by Monica C. Klempel et al. (2012) at the University of Illinois, Chicago, found that, after eight weeks, on average, the women lost a little less than 9 lbs (4 kg) in weight and a little over 2 inches (6 cm) off their waist measurement. This didn't look at the 5:2 fasting diet, though. The women consumed a combination diet of low-calorie liquid meals for six days of a week, then fasted one day a week (consuming no more than 120 calories). In addition, this was a small sample of women known to be at risk of heart disease, so they were highly motivated to lose weight, and they were only followed up for two months after the study ended.

There has been little research into the long-term effects of fasting – what evidence there is comes largely from animal studies. Probably, therefore, the medical advice would be that normal healthy, moderate eating, with plenty of fresh fruit and vegetables, is a more sustainable as well as a more enjoyable way to stay slim.

Anecdotal reports of the short-term side effects of fasting include light-headedness, lethargy, irritability, anxiety, problems sleeping, bad breath and dehydration. On a practical level, fasting may be hard to implement if, say, you have a demanding job or lifestyle, such as looking after young children. If you need to maintain concentration, too, fasting may not be right for you – feeling faint while having to drive, for example, is not a good idea. Fasting may also affect your ability to be physically active, which is, as highlighted, such an important part of maintaining a healthy weight. It can be difficult to ensure you have the recommended five portions a day of fruit and vegetables if you are fasting. Also, of course, if you have a health condition, such as diabetes or an eating disorder, or are pregnant or breastfeeding, fasting may be not just unsuitable but downright dangerous. For the averagely healthy person who is overweight or, especially, obese, the chances are that a day or two of fasting is unlikely to be harmful. It is still important, however, to seek medical advice before embarking on any such plan.

A summary and a warning

So how do I feel about fasting as a way of losing excess weight? I'm not an enthusiast. I do not think that fasting so you are perpetually hungry is the way forward for anyone – it is simply likely to make you rebound into overeating when you stop. That would lead to guilt and even more overeating in the long run. I might recommend the 5:2 option to a few patients, but would have reservations and would only do so on the proviso that they would agree to be closely supervised as they followed it.

At the start of this chapter I said that 5:2 fasting may be sensible for some people, but certainly not all. I'd like to make it clear here that it is *not* suitable for children or teenagers, who need to eat regularly because they are still growing and are more susceptible at their age than any other to eating disorders. Indeed, starting to fast may be the initial sign of anorexia or bulimia. We don't completely understand the complexities of the reasoning of youngsters who slide into these potentially lethal disorders, but it is of prime importance that we try to prevent them from doing so. Making sure that teenagers, especially girls but boys, too, are comfortable with normal eating patterns and do not become caught up in diets or fasting is of prime importance in keeping them safe from such illnesses. Suggesting that fasting might be good for them presents too much of a risk, so don't do it.

Fasting, even of the mild 5.2 type, is not for you either if you have a chronic illness that might be made worse by altering the balance of glucose and electrolytes (such as sodium, chloride, potassium and other minerals) in your blood. So, if you have diabetes, high blood pressure, heart or kidney disease, you should not attempt it without first having a long discussion with your doctor. If you already have type 2 diabetes linked to being overweight, fasting is really not for you. In short, you have to be fairly fit to fast!

Finally, if you are fasting, you must not make the mistake of trying to supplement the lack of food intake with pills. This brings up a subject that has been aggravating me for years – since 2004, to be exact. That is the year *The Lancet* published its series of articles on vitamins and supplements (Bjelakovic et al., 2004, 2007). Up until this point, I've concentrated on the benefits of exercise and healthy, rational eating, including fasting, for people who are overweight. So many people on diets reason, which seems like common sense, that if they are cutting down on foods they should at least protect themselves from harm by adding extra vitamins and minerals in the form of pills to their daily routine. I have bad news for them in the next chapter, which looks at supplement intelligence.

7

Antioxidants, vitamins, minerals and other supplement intelligence

Charles was 48 when I first met him. Around 5 feet 8 inches (1.73 m) tall, he weighed 10 stone (63.5 kg or 140 lbs). Slim to the point of being almost gaunt, flexible, twitchy, limbs always on the move even when he was seated, he was a fidget par excellence.

He had come to see me about the aches and pains he was suffering daily. He couldn't understand why he was in such trouble as he was, in his own words, 'superfit', spending an hour at least in the gym every day and 'making sure', he said, 'that I keep myself healthy by taking plenty of supplements'. He knew every detail of the advantages of consuming extra vitamins and antioxidants, so he was perplexed that he felt so miserable.

This was in 2009. I tried, gently, to persuade him that he was exercising far too hard, not resting enough and, worse, harming himself by swallowing the vast amounts of supplements that he had bought at his local gym. He didn't believe me at first, until I showed him the results of studies published three years before. He is an intelligent man, and, despite his obvious disbelief, even scorn, promised to take them home overnight. The next day he was in a rage. How could he have been so duped by all the hype about supplements when the evidence against them was so strong? How could the health media still promote them when they were doing so much harm? From that day, Charles turned into a campaigner, telling everyone he could about his epiphany. He is a healthy 52-year-old now, still exercising four days a week, a little more filled out than he was and he takes no supplements. His wife is much happier: she has a companion now who enjoys her company in the home far more than he did the gym. The local medical practice even refers patients who need practical advice on exercise to him – with great success. The gym has now given up selling supplements!

To understand why Charles became so vehement, we need to turn the clock back more than half a century, to the 1950s. That was when Dr Denham Harman (1956) unleashed on the world his 'take' on the ageing process. His research introduced to us two sets of substances with opposing actions that would become household words worldwide:

- free radicals
- antioxidants.

Free radicals, released into our tissues and organs by that life-giving molecule oxygen, caused havoc. They damaged the structure of our cells and even caused genetic damage. Allow free radicals to run loose in our bodies, Dr Harman stressed, and we would be at high risk of heart disease, cancer and a host of other life-threatening diseases.

It was a frightening discovery, but Dr Harman could reassure us. All we needed to do to stop the damage was take in plenty of 'antioxidants', which blocked the action of the free radicals. The best thing about antioxidants was that most of them were vitamins, which have to be the most innocuous of medications to take. Of course, there were plenty of vitamins in green vegetables and fresh fruit, but why not take extra, especially if you are dieting or exercising hard, just to make sure you have plenty in reserve? What possible harm could that do?

So the massive promotion of antioxidants began. Whole industries developed around them and every self-proclaimed nutritionist endorsed them. Free radicals were the villains – they had to be eliminated at all costs. Despite the fact that serious doubts were being expressed about the promotion of antioxidants by 2004 (Bjelakovic et al.) and reports of the harm they were doing were published in reputable journals in 2005 (Miller et al.) and 2007 (Bjelakovic et al.), by 2010 over half the population of the USA was still taking some form of supplement (mostly labelled as antioxidants). Americans swallow 50 billion mineral and vitamin tablets a year, which is a tribute to the massive industry making billions of dollars from them while potentially shortening their customers' lives.

I do not make this claim foolishly or lightly. My information comes from reports of large studies of people followed for years who have either taken the supplements or placebo alternatives that have been published in established and trustworthy journals such as the *Journal of the American Medical Association* and *The Lancet* (Bjelakovic, 2004, 2007; Klein et al., 2011; Miller et al., 2005; Myung et al., 2010). I'll summarize them here:

- 20 mg beta-carotene taken daily increased the rate of lung cancer in smokers by 18 per cent and their death rate by 8 per cent
- a combination of 400 IU of vitamin E with 500 mg of vitamin C given to older women with known heart disease nearly trebled their risk of dying
- vitamin E supplements increased prostate cancers by 17 per cent in previously healthy men and the higher the dose, the higher was their risk
- two reports involving many trials of multi-supplements of vitamins A, C, E, beta-carotene and selenium, intended to look at their ability to prevent cancers, found that they not only didn't prevent any form of cancer but increased, rather than decreased, mortality with one causing a rise in mortality of 6 per cent. The other was linked to a 50 per cent increase in prostate cancer – yes, 50 per cent!

It is no wonder that, on the basis of these reports, Charles became angry. What was going on?

The facts are that we need both free radicals and antioxidants to keep a balance between growth and repair and in our responses to stress, infection and cancer. To put one scientist's explanation of what went wrong simply, when a cell in any organ or tissue becomes cancerous, the neighbouring cells sense the difference in chemistry between it and them. This sets off a cascade of chemical messengers, the result of which is that the newly formed cancer cell gets the message to 'commit suicide' and destroys itself. Your natural balance between free radicals and antioxidants is crucial to this relationship.

If you overload your body with vitamins and antioxidants, this balance is disturbed. That may lead to the cancer cell being able to ignore the suicide call and continue to grow and spread. The exact mechanisms haven't yet been fully worked out, but the fact remains that surrounding cancer cells in a sea of vitamins and antioxidants must be a bad, rather than a good, idea.

I don't want to labour the argument against supplements further, except to direct you, if you want to know more, to the best book I know on the subject. It is called *The Health Delusion*, written by Glen Matten and Aidan Goggins (2012). Please read it: it is straightforward and comprehensive. Once you have, you will never want to take a multivitamin pill again.

All you have to do to satisfy your vitamin and mineral needs is eat sensibly. Eat a wide variety of foods, including fruit and vegetables, and you will fulfil all your body's needs. You don't need to pop a pill every day, with one possible exception. In recent years, a disease that we thought had vanished from the northern hemisphere has returned. In the UK, around 5 new cases a week are being reported and they could all have been prevented if people had been made aware of the risk.

Vitamin D

The disease is rickets in children and osteomalacia in adults. It is caused by failure to build up enough calcium in the bones in children and loss of bone calcium in adults. The cause is a lack of vitamin D – the vitamin that guides calcium into the skeleton.

Vitamin D is unique in that we get most of it (recent estimates are as much as 90 per cent of it) from the action of the sun on our exposed skin. If we eat well, we can absorb vitamin D from oily fish, meat, liver, eggs and foods that have been fortified with it, such as some butters, yogurts and breads, cereals, but almost certainly we won't get enough without some exposure to sunlight.

For lighter-skinned northern Europeans, most of us get enough sun from a few minutes' exposure every day from April to October, but, in the winter months, the sun never gets to a high enough angle in the sky to enable the ultraviolet light that is needed to penetrate our atmosphere so it can land on our skin. As we age, too, our skin becomes less efficient at turning the ultraviolet energy into vitamin D, so older people have less of it circulating in their blood, just at a time when they need it the most (apart from childhood) as the bones weaken with age.

Those of us who have brown skin and live in northern climes are at an even bigger disadvantage. The skin is less transparent to the ultraviolet light than lighter skin, so stronger sunlight and longer exposure to it is needed to make the same amounts of vitamin D. The tradition in some communities of covering the limbs doesn't help as it cuts down severely on the skin's ability to take advantage of what little winter sun is available.

The Canadian authorities have taken this to heart and advise Canadians to take vitamin D supplements, especially older adults, children and pregnant and nursing mothers. Osteoporosis Canada, concerned about the rising levels of bone disease among those of all ages, recommend vitamin D supplements of 400 to 1000 IU for everyone in Canada and other countries on the same latitude, even in the summertime, and for those over 50 to take double that dose. So far, the authorities in the UK have not followed suit, despite the efforts of researchers such as Dr E. Hyppönen, who, as long ago as 2007, showed that, in the UK, 87 per cent of the population fail to reach satisfactory levels of vitamin D in their blood in the winter. The figure for Scotland is 92 per cent.

There is an extra point to taking vitamin D if you are overweight or obese. Your fat cells 'mop up' much of the vitamin D in your blood and they keep it there, not even releasing it when it is needed. So, overweight people need more vitamin D than the rest of the population. That begs the question, how much vitamin D is enough?

We should be grateful to K. D. Cashman's group (2008) in Ireland who answered that question for people living in northern European latitudes. Assuming that we need at least 20 nanograms per millilitre (ng/ml) of the active form of vitamin D circulating in our blood during the wintertime to keep our bones primed with enough calcium, most people would need to take around 1000 IU of the vitamin daily from October to April, longer for those living in the far north of Scotland and the Northern Isles. In the summer, fair-skinned people who expose their arms and legs to the sun need only around four minutes of sunlight every day to avoid having to take a supplement. Those with darker skin who shade their limbs from the sun in the summertime would need to take a vitamin D supplement all the year round.

That isn't what the UK authorities recommend, though. They continue to advise that we only need to take 600 IU per day and, even then, would only recommend this for people they consider 'at risk', such as people from ethnic minorities who have very little exposure to the sun. They don't offer any advice for the rest of the public during the winter. I'm worried about that, because we have, in 2012, heard that rickets has come back to Britain, with five new cases per week being registered.

There are two last points I want to make here about taking vitamin D. The first is, please do not overdo it. As with all vitamins, more is *not* better. There is a small range of levels of vitamin D in the body that offer the optimal beneficial effect. Go below that range or above it and you can invite trouble. Taking too much vitamin D can disturb the balance of your calcium metabolism, with unpredictable consequences. Take too little and there is a risk of rickets for children or a bone-thinning disease called osteomalacia for adults.

The currently accepted optimum level of vitamin D in the blood is around 30 ng/ml. It is only in recent years, however, that researchers have managed to study enough numbers of people who have driven their levels well above this by taking extra supplements and so have learned more about its effects. Their results are rather frightening. For example, it was found in the USA that raising the levels of vitamin D in the blood in women to 50 ng/ml offered them no extra benefit in terms of their health, but was linked with a raised risk of earlier death than predicted. Other links have been found between high levels of vitamin D in the blood and prostate, oesophageal and pancreatic cancers.

The second point about vitamin D is to do with the sun. We are constantly being reminded in the media that we should not expose ourselves too much to the sun. Our life-giving star has been given the terrible reputation of causing a pandemic of skin cancers and sunbathing is dangerous, we have been told. Always put on a high-factor sun block whenever you go out in it to make sure you are not damaged by it, add a big floppy hat, a long-sleeved shirt or blouse and preferably trousers, too. Don't take any risks. The ten-fold rise in skin cancers in northern Europeans has been blamed on sunshine holidays and sunbeds. The answer, say the pundits, is to stay out of the sun's deadly rays.

Such a response is overkill, with some exceptions. It is true that excessive sunbathing in Mediterranean and subtropical latitudes will raise your risk of cancer and you should prevent the sun from burning you. Sunbeds remain a problem because most people who use them overdo their exposure and the light that they use is equivalent to summertime exposure at midday in the Mediterranean – far too strong for northern European skin. On balance, because they have been linked to an increase in the most malign of all skin cancers, melanoma, there is good evidence to support the campaign to ban sunbeds.

That said, a few minutes a day exposing your arms and legs without sunblock during a northern European summer is positively beneficial, and not harmful as long as you do not burn. You will not raise your risk of cancer – in fact, there is even evidence that if you have achieved a healthy level of vitamin D in your blood, you may even protect yourself from bowel cancer.

So, enjoy what summer sunshine you can get if you are in the British Isles and don't be afraid to spend a few minutes in it, even in the midday sun, without sunblock. The odd thing about deriving your vitamin D from the sun is that, once you have achieved normal levels of the vitamin in your blood, your skin will shut down production of it until you start to need more, even if you continue to expose yourself to the sun. Lifeguards on Pacific beaches, whose light-coloured skins are massively exposed to, and certainly not maximally protected against, ultraviolet light, have vitamin D levels of only around 30 ng/ml in their blood – the optimal level, achieved naturally.

A final note on taking supplements

To summarize, if you are thinking of taking any supplement at all, the only one that has good scientific evidence behind it is vitamin D, but you must not overdo it. There is no need to take a supplement if the level of vitamin D in your blood is around 30 ng/ml. If you are doubtful about your vitamin D status, please talk it over with your doctor. Checking the level involves a simple test and will help you to come to a safe decision as to whether or not to take it, at least during wintertime. That is particularly true if you are trying to lose weight by dieting as some restrictive diets may be deficient in vitamin D and so you may develop a deficiency as a result without realizing it. If you are eating a normal variety of foods, that is much less likely to happen.

8

Surgery for obesity

It is 25 years since the death of the morbidly obese young woman I wrote about earlier in the section on overweight and obese children in Chapter 2. If she had been alive today she would have been offered intensive management of her obesity and been considered for bariatric surgery. With the expertise in surgery for the morbidly obese that is available today, I am sure, if she and her family had accepted it and followed the advice, the outcome would have been very different and she would still be with us.

Someone is defined as obese if he or she has a body mass index (BMI) of more than 30 (about 25 per cent above the normal weight for height) and morbidly obese if the BMI is above 40 (which is double the normal weight for height). In effect, being morbidly obese means carrying more than 10 stone (64 kg or 140 lbs) around with you all the time. Many people on the list for bariatric surgery are even heavier than that.

Faced with patients who are so overweight, doctors first try to get them to lose weight by means other than surgery. At best, however, eating less and exercising more will only produce a weight loss of around 11 lbs (5 kg) in the first year – even if the patient is still able to move about enough to use up the energy taken in from a meagre amount of food.

The effects of drugs to lessen appetite are limited, too, producing only modest weight loss for a few weeks, then tailing off. They also have serious side effects. For example, orlistat often causes digestive upsets, rimonabant has been linked with severe depression and sibutramine can cause abnormalities in the heart rhythm. This is the first and only mention of slimming drugs in the book, which is deliberate. That is because they rarely succeed and cause so many problems that few specialists in obesity use them regularly, except in very exceptional cases.

So, for people who are excessively obese and so ill because of it that their life expectancy is very short, bariatric surgery is their only option. Surgeons never take the prospect of such an operation lightly and nor should their patients.

'Bariatrics' is the medical specialty that concentrates on obesity and its related problems. Bariatric surgery aims to change someone's life permanently. It has two aims:

- to restrict the amount of food that can be eaten
- to prevent food that is eaten from being digested and absorbed.

The first is achieved by gastric banding, in which, using keyhole surgery, a tight silicone band is placed around the upper part of the stomach. The aim is to make the person feel full after eating much less food than they have been used to. The width of the band can be adjusted after the operation by injecting material into, or withdrawing material from, a 'port' under the skin of the abdomen that is connected to the band.

The second aim gives people the choice of several operations, all of which involve diverting food away from the stomach, bypassing the first part of the digestive process. In effect, this stops much of the food that has been eaten from being absorbed. The commonest form of gastric bypass is the Roux-en-Y operation, which shuts off most of the stomach from the rest of the intestine, leaving only a small pouch that is then joined up to the small intestine.

Sounds tricky? There is a much trickier operation called biliopancreatic diversion, in which the lower third of the stomach is removed and the upper part that is left is joined to the small intestine much lower down. It involves removing a substantial length of small intestine, too.

It is a sign of how attitudes have changed since the year 2000 that 261 bariatric operations were performed in the UK that year, while the current annual score is more than 8000 (although more than 1000 of them are band adjustments, they count as separate operations). This 30-fold rise is largely due to the recognition that other treatments, such as diets and exercise, have failed miserably in the treatment of the obese and morbidly obese and to the fact that the UK's NHS has understood that an effective method of managing serious obesity will, in the long run, reduce the costs of its consequences, such as the care of diabetes, high blood pressure, stroke, heart failure, heart attack and multiple organ failure.

Do the operations work? If they do, who should be offered them? Are there serious complications?

The short answers to all these questions are that they do, they are open to morbidly obese adults and those whose BMI is 35 to 40 so they don't qualify on that basis, but who have illnesses such as diabetes and high blood pressure, which is the metabolic syndrome mentioned in Chapter 5. The success of the operations, however, has to be weighed up against a series of problems that can arise from the surgery.

Here are the figures (first published in the USA), so you can judge for yourself. By 2004, H. Buchwald had reviewed 25 studies involving 3873 people who had had a gastric band fitted. They lost an average of 4 stone 6 lbs (28 kg or 62 lbs), which is impressive, but, more importantly, 48 per cent of them had also lost their diabetes, 59 per cent had returned to normal blood cholesterol levels and 71 per cent had lowered their blood pressure to normal or near-normal levels. Probably best of all, 68 per cent of the people involved in the study had lost their sleep apnoea, too – the condition that killed my young woman patient. There have been many more studies of the outcomes of gastric band operations since this one and all of the results point in the same direction.

Gastric bypass operations have produced even better results. Buchwald brought together 44 studies of such operations given to a total of 7074 patients. They lost a mean of 6 stone 11 lbs (43 kg or 95 lbs). Also, 84 per cent of them lost their diabetes, 97 per cent lost their high blood cholesterol scores and, in a massive 95 per cent of cases, the sleep apnoea either disappeared or was considerably reduced.

A comparison of the results of gastric band v. gastric bypass operations for 'super-morbidly' obese patients (having a BMI of over 50) came out strongly in favour of the bypass option, which led to much greater weight loss, had fewer instances of complications and further operations, a spectacular cure rate for diabetes (100 per cent of the bypass patients lost their diabetes) and sleep apnoea (a fall from 54 to 8 per cent).

Neither operation is without problems. Bands can slip, migrate, leak or cause allergic reactions and infections – all of which can threaten life. Because the gastric bypass operation is more complicated, involving cutting into and joining up areas of stomach and bowel, staple lines can come apart and suture lines can leak or cause blockages. Around one in six people develops nutritional deficiencies after a gastric bypass operation that need to be managed in the long term. Considering the difficulties of operating on people with so much fatty tissue, the number of deaths from bands is tiny (10 patients in a series of 17,644). There are more deaths after bypass operations (16 in 1000 in the 30 days after laparoscopic surgery), but these numbers are astonishingly low when you consider that the bypass patients are almost always much more overweight than those selected for gastric band operations.

Gastric bands work best for people with BMIs from 35 to 39, aged from 15 to 39 years, who increase their physical activity and change their eating habits after surgery. It is not so successful for people who have higher BMIs, few of whom achieve adequate weight loss after the surgery.

In 2008, the UK's National Institute for Health and Care Excellence (NICE) set guidelines for bariatric surgery. People will only qualify if their BMI is 40 or more or if, with a BMI from 35 to 40, they have poorly controlled diabetes and/or high blood pressure. They must also already have tried, for at least six months, and failed to lose weight using all the conventional treatments and advice. Further, they must agree to receive intensive management from a specialist obesity service, be fit for anaesthesia and surgery and commit themselves to long-term follow-up monitoring after the operation. They should also be prepared to have further surgery afterwards to remove the excess loose skin that will inevitably form an 'apron' over the abdomen after they will have lost more than 5 stone (32 kg or 70 lbs). The surgery is thus actually called an 'apronectomy'. Last of all, they must be mentally strong enough to work on reducing the various possible costs of the consequences of not improving the management of their weight after surgery. They include the long-term care of the complications of continuing diabetes, such as possible blindness, kidney failure and amputations, as well as heart failure, heart attack, stroke and, eventually, multiple organ failure that are accentuated by diabetes. Those who are not diabetic but severely obese are also at high risk of these latter eventualities. Thus, people who are massively overweight face huge health-related, social and financial struggles as they enter their later middle age.

Bariatric surgery is the fastest and most successful way to lose excess weight, but it is not a standalone treatment. It won't be successful if those having it don't accept that they have been given the chance of a new life, casting off one that would have been much shorter without it. They also need to start, then continue, on that second life with a different approach to eating and exercise. After years of overeating and underexercising it is not possible to make these changes without professional help. That is the reason for the NICE guidelines. The Appendix summarizes the advice of the organization that has had the most to do with the complications of obesity – the British Heart Foundation.

Appendix
Dietary intelligence

By now you will understand why I have left dietary advice until last. All through this book there has been a theme – that exercise is the key and eating is part of one's joys in life, not a medication. So, calorie-counting and the measuring of portions have not featured at all.

If you eat what you need and exercise enough to use up the energy latent in your food, you will not be obese and your weight will not vary significantly. If you are overweight, you can use any exercise that you enjoy or that you can learn to enjoy (slothdom can be hard to give up) to lose the excess, provided that you don't overcompensate for the energy you use up by then gorging yourself.

It is self-evident, however, that simply saying eat healthily and don't take in more than that required for your energy output is neglecting one side of the eating–exercise equation. We still need evidence-based guidance on the details of what and how much to eat. For me, the best guidance comes from the experts who have most to gain from our population eating sensibly – the British Heart Foundation (BHF). The organ most at risk from uncontrolled obesity is the heart, so the BHF has spent much time and relied on the expertise of those who know to work out how to get the balance right. So, here is my summary of the BHF's advice on obesity to the UK's GPs and their patients.

First, assess your dietary intake. That isn't so easy unless you keep a diary in which you write, at the time, what you are eating or drinking. Don't forget to include any alcoholic drinks – they can hide surprisingly high energy content. Diaries reveal more about you than you might think. For example, they will help you answer the following questions.

- Are you a regular meal eater or do you snack?
- Do you prefer sweet or savoury foods?
- What foods do you actively dislike?
- What foods do you find difficult to resist?
- What foods trigger binge eating?
- What is your typical portion size? (A photograph would help your doctor.)
- How do you eat at work – packed lunches, the pub, a canteen?
- Who does the cooking at home and shops for food? Does he or she provide ready meals or traditional meals?

How you answer these questions gives an insight into where your eating problems may lie and how they can be adjusted. You may not realize quite how much you eat every day if you don't create a written diary and a question and answer page. When you sit down with your doctor or nutritionist or nurse, the ramifications of the answers may shock you.

Take a few examples from the list – starting with portion size. Many people can successfully lose weight simply by reducing their portion sizes. Eating more slowly (remember the ghrelin and leptin relationship in Chapters 1 and 5) makes it easier for you to do so without feeling pangs of hunger. To take some simple examples, you only need three tablespoons of cereal for breakfast and when you are eating potatoes, two egg-sized ones are enough. Two heaped tablespoons of rice is enough for a single portion.

As for your meal pattern, structured mealtimes and home-cooked food help you to choose less energy dense foods, rather than buying ready meals full of fats and sugars. Note that skipping meals on odd days rarely helps to reduce your overall energy intake, except, apparently, when you are following Dr Mosley's 5:2 fast (see Chapter 6).

If circumstances force you to snack, then choose your snack carefully. Fruit, fresh or dried (incidentally, don't swallow dried fruit whole, always chew it well, as otherwise it may swell in your gut and cause an obstruction), raw vegetables, yogurts, and low-sugar breakfast cereals, such as muesli or porridge, made with semi-skimmed milk, are good choices.

The British Heart Foundation gives very specific advice on fats, carbohydrates and proteins. It stresses that fat gives us 9 calories per gram, while carbohydrates and proteins each give only 4. So, look at food labels for foods containing under 3 g of fat per 100 g (a little under 1 oz per 3½ oz) and choose low-fat substitutes when you can. Try to limit the fat you use in cooking, too. Your carbohydrate needs are covered by bread, pasta, potatoes and rice, which should form the basis of your meals. You can fulfil your protein needs from meat, poultry (without the skin) low-fat dairy products and pulses.

Best of all is to eat plenty of fruit and vegetables. They provide very few calories, yet add bulk to your meal, giving you the feeling of fullness that stops you eating too much. They are also rich in vitamins and plant chemicals that may protect your heart and your bodily systems from other diseases.

There is one don't and, even then, it is not a complete no-no. The BHF experts do ask those wanting to lose weight to avoid cakes, biscuits, chocolate and sweets, as they are energy dense, but they are not complete killjoys. They say that eating them occasionally, as special treats, will not ruin weeks or months of your eating discipline.

The main message remains, however. Get active and get a life – it is the only one you have.

References

ActiveScotland: www.activescotland.org.uk

Al-Shayji, I. A. R., Caslake, M. J. and Gill, J. M. R. (2012) 'Effects of moderate exercise on VLDL1 and intralipid kinetics in overweight/obese middle-aged men', *American Journal of Physiology-Endocrinology and Metabolism*, 302(3): e349–55.

Almond, C. S. D., Shin, A. Y., Fortescue, E. B., Mannix, R. C., Wypij, D. et al. (2005) 'Hyponatremia among runners in the Boston Marathon', *New England Journal of Medicine*, 352(15): 1550–6, 14 April.

Andersen, L. B., Schnor, P., Schroll, M. and Hein, H. O. (2000) 'All-cause mortality associated with physical activity during leisure time, work, sports, and cycling to work', *Archives of Internal Medicine*, 160: 1621–8.

Archenti, A. and Pasqualinotto, L. (2008), 'Childhood obesity: the epidemic of the third millenium', *ACTA BIOMED*, 79: 151–5.

Bauman, A. E, Reis, R. S., Sallis, J. F., Wells, J. C., Loos, R. J. F. and Martin, B. W. (2012) 'Correlates of physical activity: Why are some people physically active and others not?', *The Lancet*, 380(9838): 258–71, 21 July.

Bell, A. C., Ge, K. and Popkin, B. M. (2002) 'The road to obesity or the path to prevention: Motorized transportation and obesity in China', *Obesity Research*, 10(4): 277–83.

Bjelakovic, G., Nikolova, D., Gluud, L. L., Simonetti, R. G. and Gluud, C. (2007) 'Mortality in randomized trials of antioxidant supplements for primary and secondary prevention: Systematic review and meta-analysis', *The Journal of the American Medical Association*, 297(8): 842–57, 28 February.

Bjelakovic, G., Nikolova, D., Simonetti, R. G. and Gluud, C. (2004) 'Antioxidant supplements for prevention of gastrointestinal cancers: A systematic review and meta-analysis', *The Lancet*, 364(9441): 1219–28, 2 October.

Blair, S. (2009) 'Physical inactivity: The biggest public health problem of the 21st century', *British Journal of Sports Medicine*, 43: 1–2.

Buchwald, H., Avidor, Y., Braunwald, E., Jensen, M. D., Pories, W., Fahrbach, K. and Schoelles, K. (2004) 'Bariatric surgery: A systematic review and meta-analysis', *The Journal of the American Medical Association*, 292(14): 1724–37, 13 October.

Cashman, K. D., Hill, T. R., Lucey, A. J., Taylor, N., Seamans, K. M., Muldowney, S. et al. (2008) 'Estimation of the dietary requirement for vitamin D in healthy adults', *American Journal of Clinical Nutrition*, 88(6): 1535–42, December.

Coghlan, A. (2010) 'Food, not flab, makes obesity a killer', *New Scientist*, 205(2751): 8–9, 10 March.

Coghlan, A. (2012) 'The workout pill: Why exercise is the best medicine', *New Scientist*, 215(2879): 38–41, 29 August.

Cohen, D. (2012) 'The truth about sports drinks', *British Medical Journal*, 345: e4737, 19 July.

de Geus, E. J. and de Moor, M. H. (2011) 'Genes, exercise and psychological factors', in Bouchard, C. and Hoffman, E. P. (eds) *Genetic and Molecular Aspects of Sports Performance*. Oxford: Blackwell, 294–305.

Dolan, P. and Kavetsos, G. (2012) ' Educational interventions are unlikely to work because obese people aren't unhappy enough to lose weight', *British Medical Journal*, 345: e8487, 26 June.

Flegal, K. M., Carroll, M. D., Kit, B. K., and Ogden, C. L. (2012) 'Prevalence of obesity and trends in the distribution of body mass index among US adults, 1999–2010', *Journal of the American Medical Association*, 307(5): 491–7.

Floegel, A. and Pischon, T. (2012) 'Low carbohydrate–high protein diets', *British Medical Journal*, Editorial, 344: e3801, 19 June.

Frayling, T. (2012) 'Are the causes of obesity primarily environmental?: No', *British Medical Journal*, 345: e5844, 11 September.

'Global Burden of Disease Study' (2012) *The Lancet*, 380(9859): 2053–60, 15 December.

Harman, D. (1956) 'Aging: A theory based on free radical and radiation chemistry', *Journal of Gerontolology*, 11(3): 298–300, July.

Harvie, M. N., Pegington, M., Mattson, M. P., Frystyk, J., Dillon, B. et al. (2011) 'The effects of intermittent or continuous energy restriction on weight loss and metabolic disease risk markers: A randomized trial in young overweight women', *International Journal of Obesity*, 35: 714–727, May.

Heshka, S. A., Atkinson, J. W., Atkinson, R. L., Greenway, F. L., Hill, J. O., Phinney, S. D., Kolotkin, R. L., Miller-Kovach, K. and Pi-Sunyer, F. X. (2003) 'Weight loss with self-help compared with a structured commercial program: A randomized trial', *Journal of the American Medical Association*, 289(14): 1792–8.

Hill, A. J. (2004) 'Does dieting make you fat?', *British Journal of Nutrition*, 92(1): S15–S18.

Hyppönen, E. and Power, C. (2007) 'Hypovitaminosis D in British adults at age 45 y: Nationwide cohort study of dietary and lifestyle predictors', *American Journal of Clinical Nutrition*, 85(3): 860–8.

Japan Times, The (2012) 'Inactivity amid nuclear crisis leaving Fukushima children out of shape', *The Japan Times*, 26 December.

Kimm, S. Y., Glynn, N. W., Obarzanek, E., Kriska, A. M., Daniels, S. R., Barton, B. A. and Liu, K. (2005) 'Relation between the changes in physical activity and body-mass index during adolescence: A multicentre longitudinal study', *The Lancet* 366(9482): 301–7, 23 July.

Klein, E. A., Thompson, I. M., Tangen, C. M., Crowley, J. J. Lucia, M. S. et al. (2011) 'Vitamin E and the risk of prostate cancer: The selenium and vitamin E cancer prevention trial (SELECT)', *The Journal of the American Medical Association*, 306(14): 1549–56, 12 October.

Klempel, M. C., Kroeger, C. M., Bhutani, S., Trepanowski, J. F. and Varady, K. A. (2012) 'Intermittent fasting combined with calorie restriction is effective for weight loss and cardio-protection in obese women', *Nutrition Journal*, 11: 98, 21 November.

Kmietowicz, Z. (2013) 'Multidisciplinary teams are needed throughout UK to manage obesity', *British Medical Journal*, 346: e8679, 29 May.

Krustrup, P., Aagaard, P., Nybo, L., Petersen, J., Mohr, M., et al. (2010) 'Recreational football as a health-promoting activity: A topical review', *Scandinavian Journal of Medical Science*, Sports Supplement, 1: 1–13.

Lagiou, P., Sandin, S., Lof, M., Trichopoulos, D., Adami, H.-O. and Weiderpass, E. (2012) 'Low carbohydrate-high protein diet and incidence of cardiovascular diseases in Swedish women: Prospective cohort study', *British Medical Journal*, 344: e4026, 26 June.

Lee, I.-M., Shiroma, E., Lobelo, F. et al. 'Effect of physical inactivity on major non-communicable diseases worldwide: An analysis of burden of disease and life expectancy', The Lancet Physical Activity Series Working Group, *The Lancet* 380(9838): 219–29, 21 July.

Martinez-Gonzales, M.A., Martinez, J. A., Hu, F. B. et al. (1999) 'Physical inactivity, sedentary lifestyle and obesity in the European Union', *International Journal of Obesity*, 23: 1192–201.

Matten, G. and Goggins, A. (2012) *The Health Delusion: How to achieve exceptional health in the 21st century*. London: Hay House.

Miller III, F. R., Pastor-Barriuso, R., Dalal, D., Riemersma, R. A., Appel, L. J. and Guallar, E. (2005) 'Meta-analysis: High-dosage vitamin E supplementation may increase all-cause mortality', *Annals of Internal Medicine*, 142(1): 37–46, 4 January.

Mosley, M. (2012) 'The 5:2 diet: Can it help you lose weight and live longer?', *The Telegraph*, 16 August.

Myung, S.-K., Kim, Y., Ju, W., Choi, H. J. and Bae, W. K. (2010) 'Effects of antioxidant supplements on cancer prevention: Meta-analysis of randomized controlled trials', *Annals of Oncology*, 21(1): 166–79.

Neel, J. (1962) 'Diabetes mellitus: A "thrifty" genotype rendered detrimental by "progress"?', *American Journal of Human Genetics*, 14: 353–62.

Noakes, T. (2012) *Waterlogged: The serious problem of overhydration in endurance sports*. Champaign, IL: Human Kinetics.

OECD (2012) 'Obesity update 2012', OECD, Paris.

Ogden, C. L., Carroll, M. D., Kit, B. K. and Flegal, K. M. (2012) 'Prevalence of obesity and trends in body mass index among US children and adolescents, 1999–2010', *Journal of the American Medical Association*, 307(5): 483–90.

Parkes, A., Sweeting, H. and Wight, D. (2012) 'Growing Up in Scotland: Overweight, obesity and activity', Scottish Government, Edinburgh.

Ravussin, E., Valencia, M. E, Esparza J., Bennett, P. H. and Schulz, L. O.

(1994) 'Effects of a traditional lifestyle on obesity in Pima Indians', *Diabetes Care*, 17(9): 1067–74.

Robert Wood Johnson Foundation (2012) 'Consumption of sports drinks by children and adolescents: A research review', June, *Healthy Eating Research*, Robert Wood Johnson Foundation, Princeton, NJ.

Rosenbaum, M. and Leibel, R. L. (2010) 'Adaptive thermogenesis in humans', *International Journal of Obesity*, 34: S47–S55, October.

Westphal, V. K. and Smith, J. E. (1996) 'Overeaters anonymous: Who goes and who succeeds?', *Eating Disorders* 4(2): 160–70.

Woollett, K. and Maguire, E. A. (2011) 'Acquiring "the Knowledge" of London's layout drives structural brain changes', *Current Biology*, 21(24): 2109–14.

Index